This Journal Belongs To

_____

My Starting Measurements

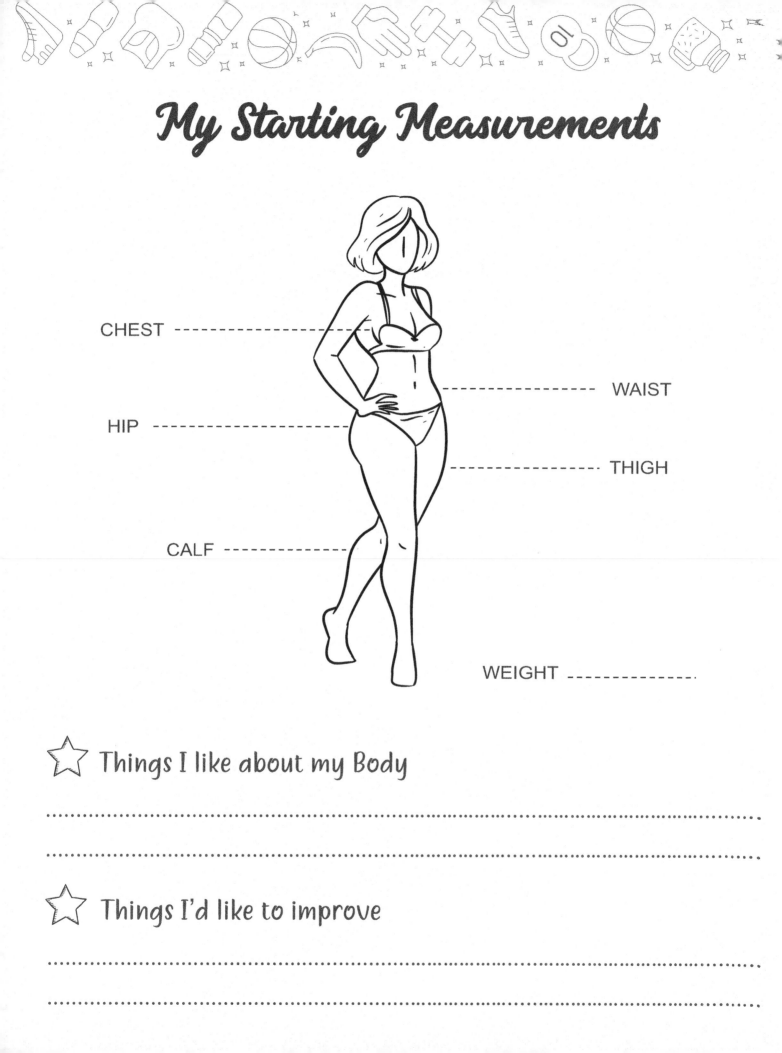

CHEST - - - - - - - - - - - - - - - - - -

WAIST - - - - - - - - - - - - - - -

HIP - - - - - - - - - - - - - - -

THIGH - - - - - - - - - - - - - -

CALF - - - - - - - - - - -

WEIGHT - - - - - - - - - - - - -

☆ Things I like about my Body

....

....

☆ Things I'd like to improve

....

....

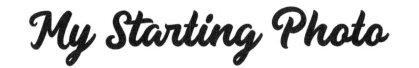

My Starting Photo

Glue in a photo of yourself, not the perfect one!
So you can look back at it at the end of your journey to be amazed!

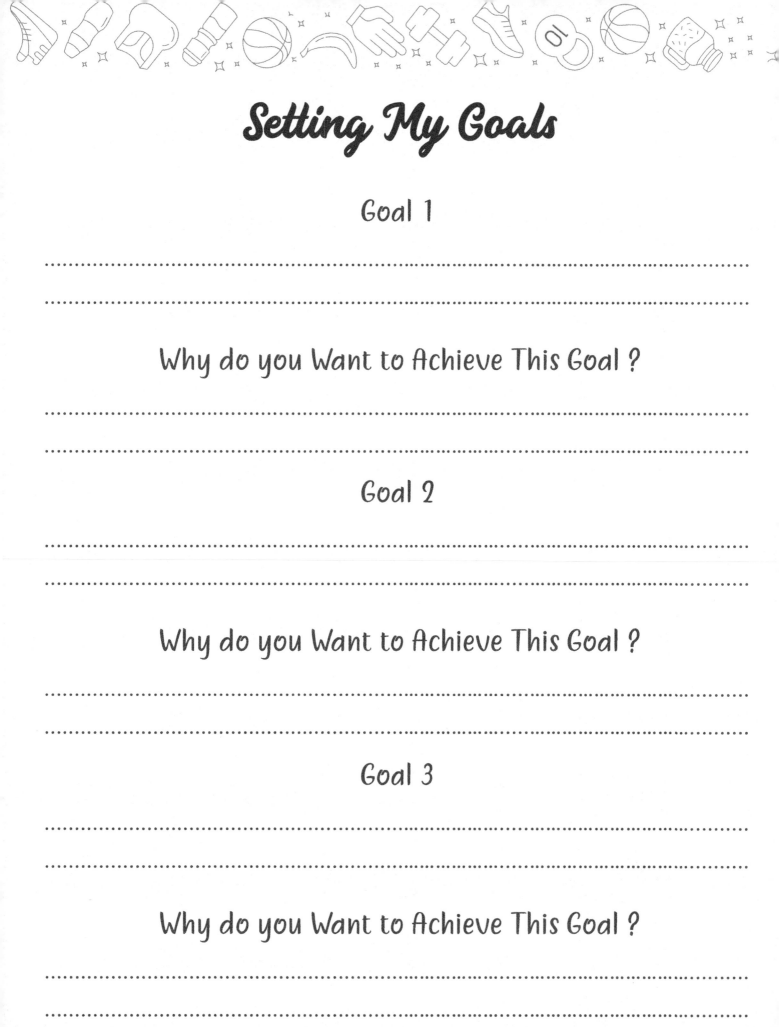

Setting My Goals

Goal 1

....
....

Why do you Want to Achieve This Goal ?

....
....

Goal 2

....
....

Why do you Want to Achieve This Goal ?

....
....

Goal 3

....
....

Why do you Want to Achieve This Goal ?

....
....

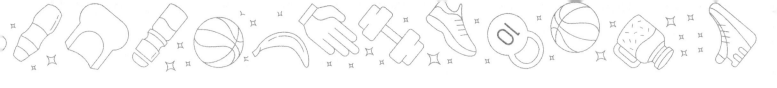

Progress Tracker

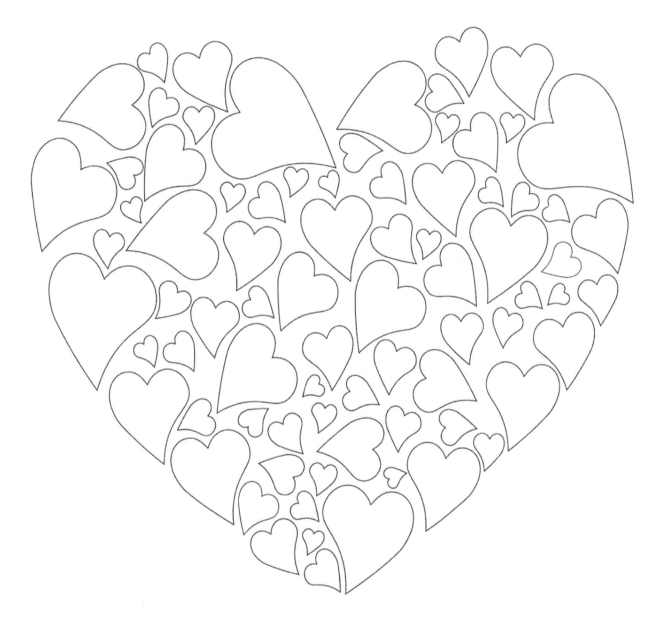

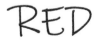 COLOR YOUR DAY <

RED
If Completed

Yellow
If Completed
partially
(e.g. missed out fitness log,
water intake etc.)

Black
If Skipped

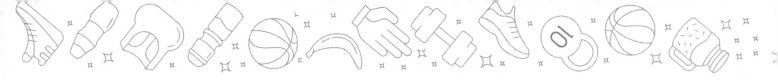

Weekly Check-in

Weekly Goals

☐ _____
_____

☐ _____
_____

☐ _____
_____

Measurements

CHEST	
WAIST	
HIPS	
THIGH	
CALF	
WEIGHT	

Good Habits to Build

_____
_____
_____
_____
_____

Bad Habits to Cut

_____
_____
_____
_____
_____

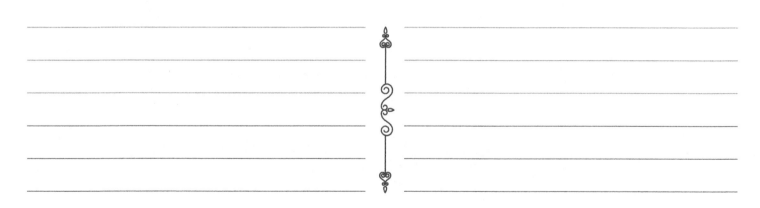

How I'm Feeling

_____
_____
_____
_____

Reasons to keep Going

_____
_____
_____
_____

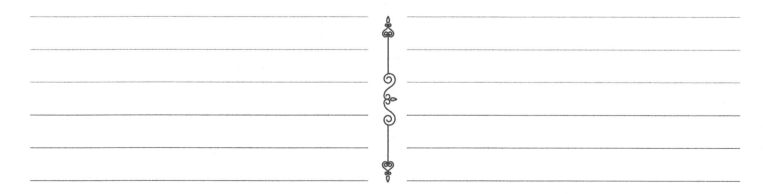

Date: ....   **Weight:** ....

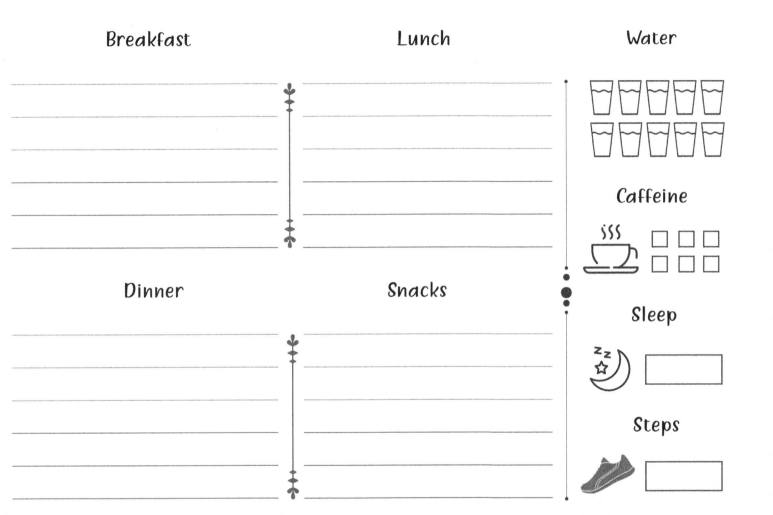

Breakfast	Lunch	Water

Dinner   **Snacks**

Caffeine

Sleep

Steps

ACTIVITY/EXERCISE	AMOUNT	NOTES

My mood is   **How to make tomorrow better**

Date:................... Weight:.................

Breakfast

_____
_____
_____
_____

Lunch

_____
_____
_____
_____

Water

☐☐☐☐☐
☐☐☐☐☐

Caffeine

☐☐☐
☐☐☐

Dinner

_____
_____
_____
_____

Snacks

_____
_____
_____
_____

Sleep

[____]

Steps

[____]

ACTIVITY/EXERCISE	AMOUNT	NOTES

My Mood is

_____
_____
_____

How to make tomorrow better

_____
_____
_____

Date:............... Weight:...............

Breakfast

_____
_____
_____
_____
_____

Lunch

_____
_____
_____
_____
_____

Water

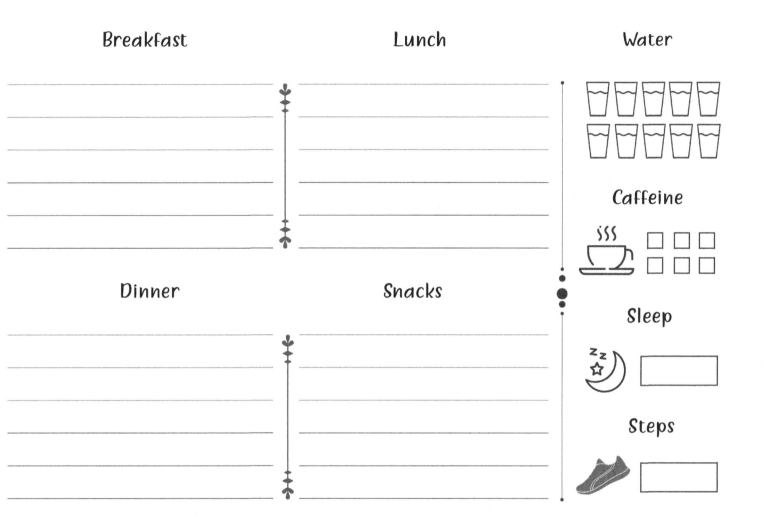

Dinner

_____
_____
_____
_____
_____

Snacks

_____
_____
_____
_____
_____

Caffeine

Sleep

Steps

ACTIVITY/EXERCISE	AMOUNT	NOTES

My Mood is

_____
_____

How to make tomorrow better

_____
_____

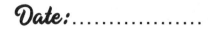

Date:................. **Weight:**.................

Breakfast

_____
_____
_____
_____
_____

Lunch

_____
_____
_____
_____
_____

Water

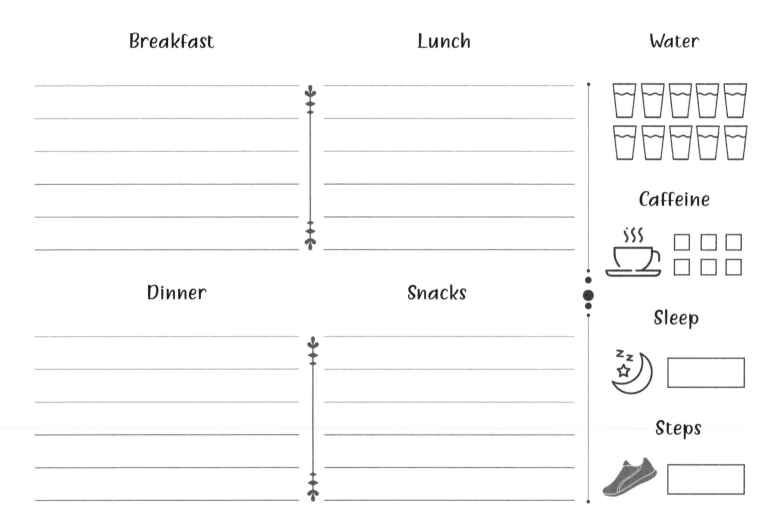

Caffeine

Dinner

_____
_____
_____
_____

Snacks

_____
_____
_____
_____

Sleep

Steps

ACTIVITY/EXERCISE	AMOUNT	NOTES

My Mood is

_____
_____
_____

How to make tomorrow better

_____
_____
_____

Date: ....   **Weight:** ....

Breakfast	Lunch	Water

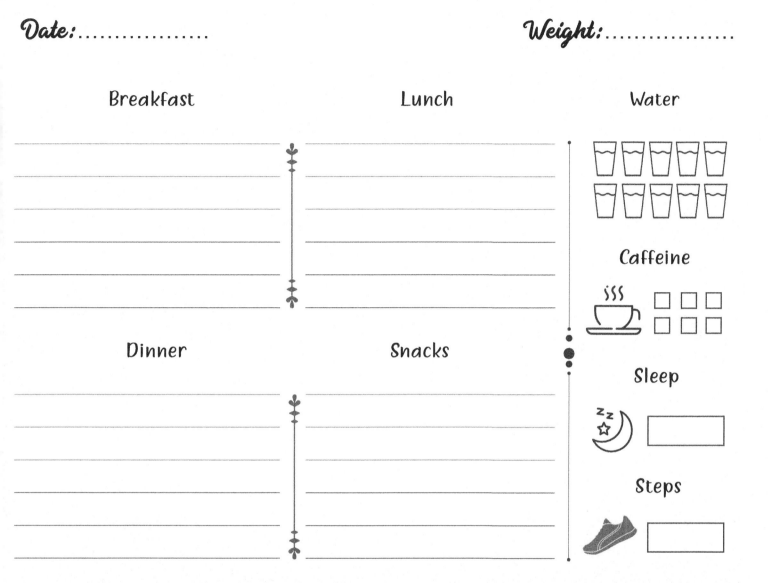

Dinner   Snacks

Caffeine

Sleep

Steps

ACTIVITY/EXERCISE	AMOUNT	NOTES

My Mood is

How to make tomorrow better

Date: ....   **Weight:** ....

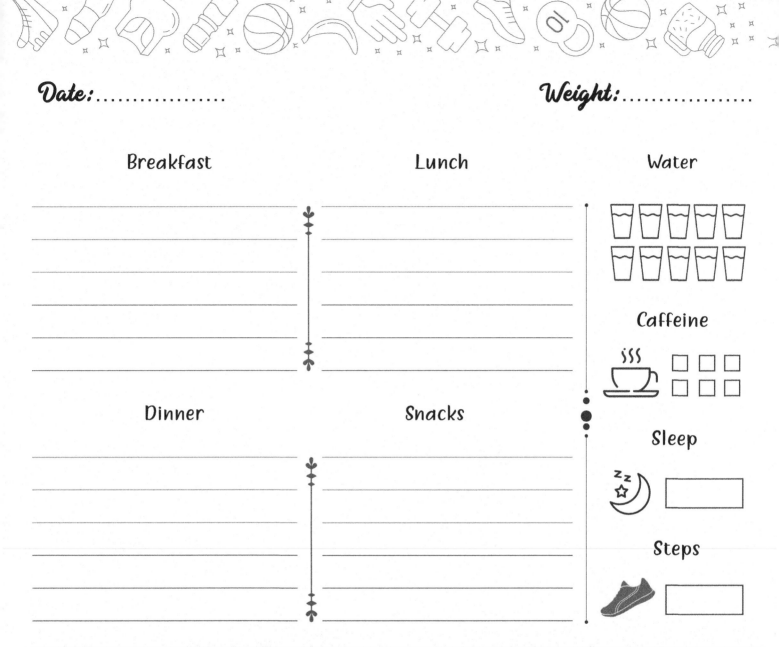

Breakfast

Lunch

Water

Dinner

Snacks

Caffeine

Sleep

Steps

ACTIVITY/EXERCISE	AMOUNT	NOTES

My Mood is

How to make tomorrow better

Date: .... Weight: ....

Breakfast

Lunch

Water

Dinner

Snacks

Caffeine

Sleep

Steps

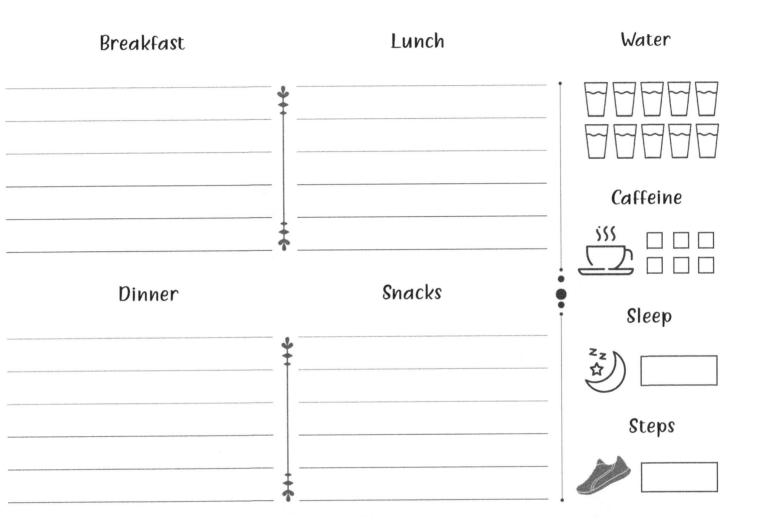

ACTIVITY/EXERCISE	AMOUNT	NOTES

My Mood is

How to make tomorrow better

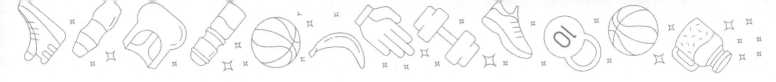

Weekly Check-in

Weekly Goals

- [ ]
- [ ]
- [ ]

Measurements

CHEST	
WAIST	
HIPS	
THIGH	
CALF	
WEIGHT	

Good Habits to Build

Bad Habits to Cut

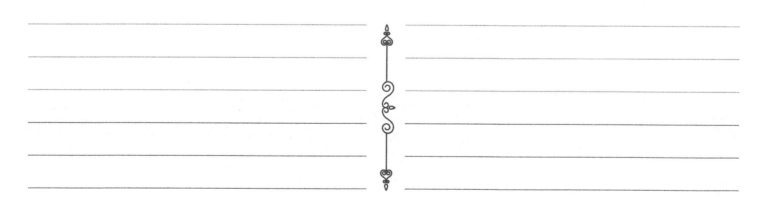

How I'm Feeling

Reasons to keep Going

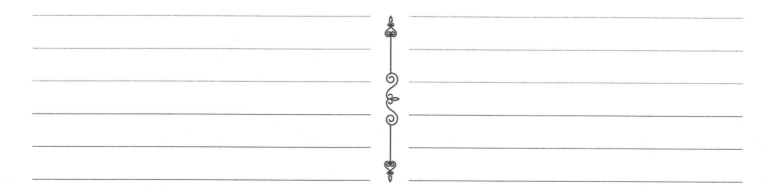

Date: ....

Weight: ....

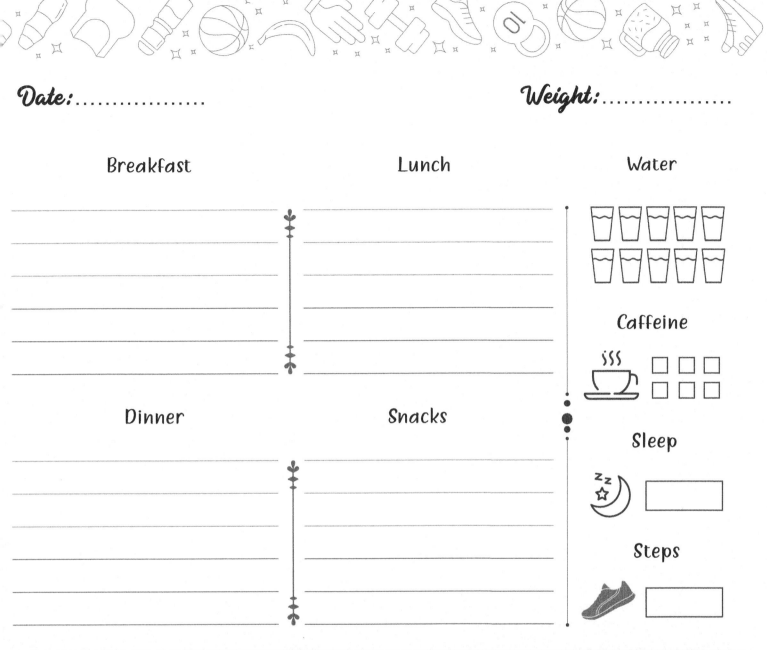

Breakfast

Lunch

Water

Dinner

Snacks

Caffeine

Sleep

Steps

ACTIVITY/EXERCISE	AMOUNT	NOTES

My Mood is

How to make tomorrow better

Date:.................   Weight:.................

Breakfast   Lunch   Water

_____   _____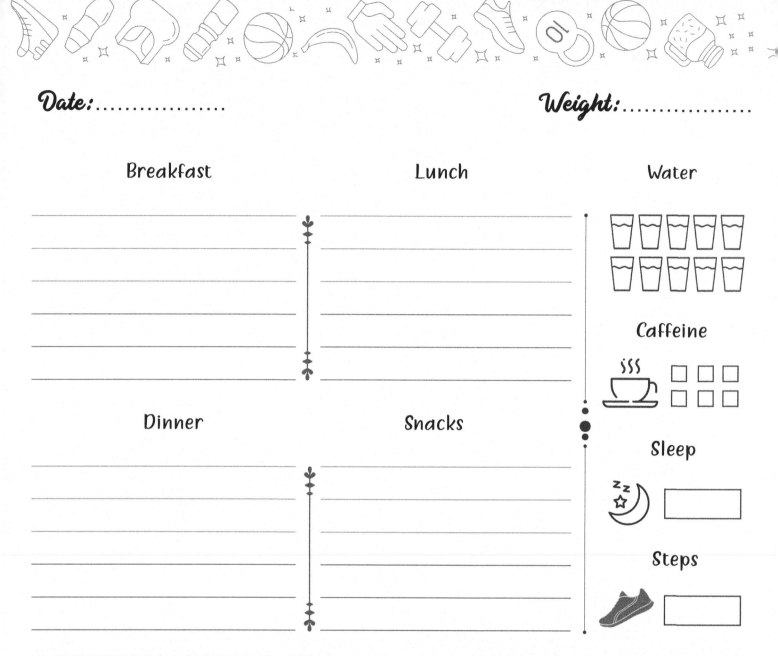

_____   _____

_____   _____   Caffeine

_____   _____

Dinner   Snacks   Sleep

_____   _____

_____   _____   Steps

_____   _____

_____   _____

ACTIVITY/EXERCISE	AMOUNT	NOTES

My Mood is   How to make tomorrow better

_____   _____

_____   _____

_____   _____

Date: ....   Weight: ....

Breakfast

_____
_____
_____
_____
_____

Lunch

_____
_____
_____
_____
_____

Water

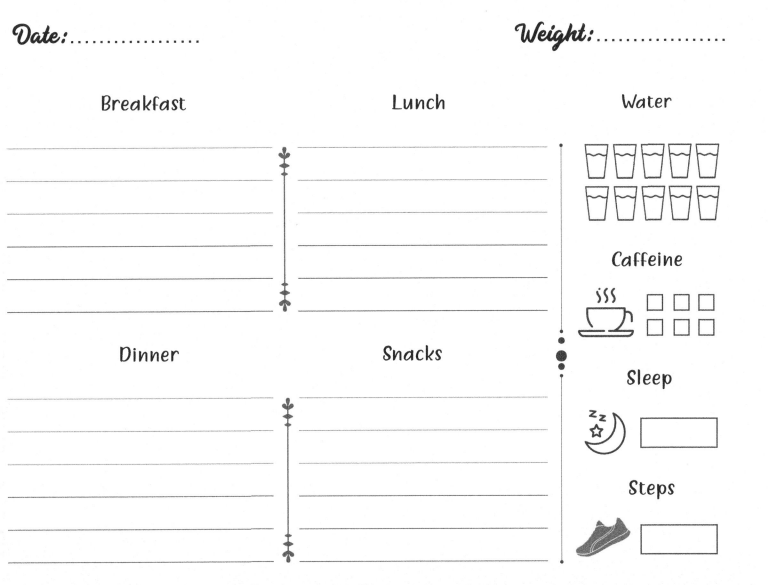

Caffeine

Sleep

Steps

Dinner

_____
_____
_____
_____
_____

Snacks

_____
_____
_____
_____
_____

ACTIVITY/EXERCISE	AMOUNT	NOTES

My Mood is

_____
_____
_____

How to make tomorrow better

_____
_____
_____

Date:................   Weight:..................

Breakfast   Lunch   Water

_____   _____
_____   _____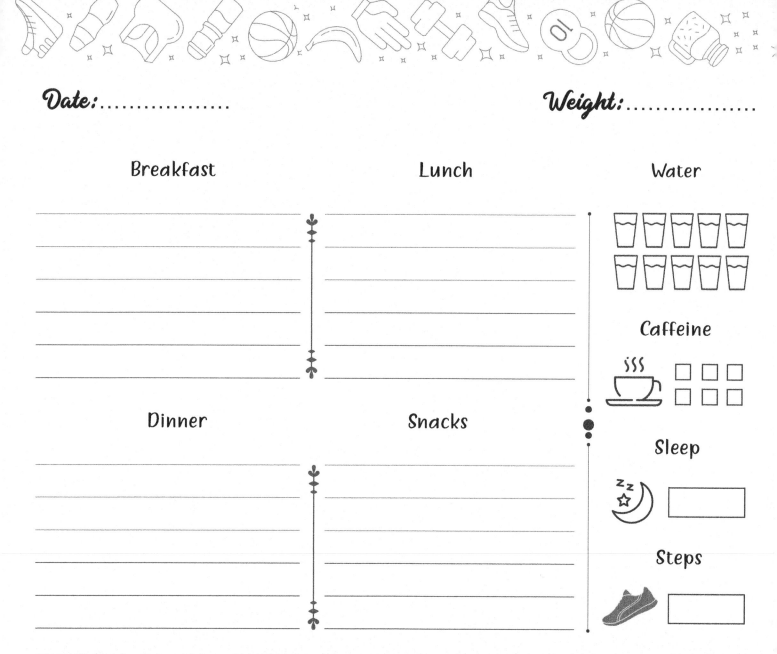
_____   _____
_____   _____   Caffeine
_____   _____

Dinner   Snacks   Sleep

_____   _____
_____   _____
_____   _____   Steps
_____   _____

ACTIVITY/EXERCISE	AMOUNT	NOTES

My Mood is   How to make tomorrow better

_____   _____
_____   _____
_____   _____

Date: .... Weight: ....

Breakfast

_____
_____
_____
_____

Lunch

_____
_____
_____
_____

Water

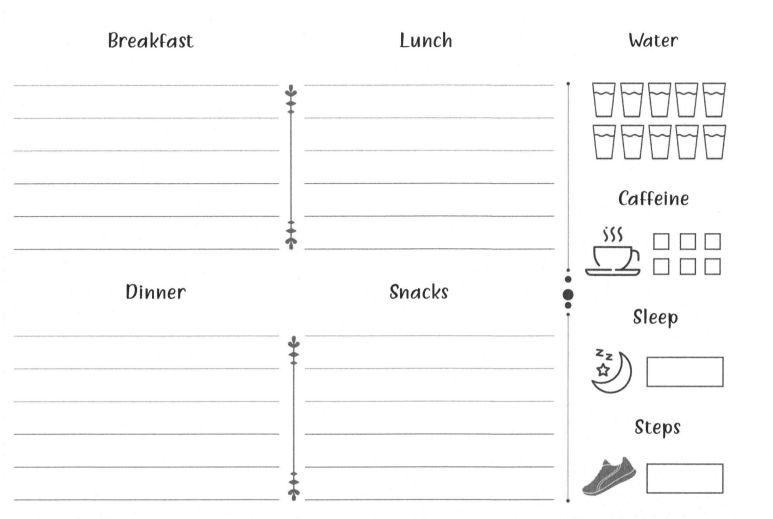

Caffeine

Sleep

Steps

Dinner

_____
_____
_____
_____

Snacks

_____
_____
_____
_____

ACTIVITY/EXERCISE	AMOUNT	NOTES

My Mood is

_____
_____

How to make tomorrow better

_____
_____

Date: ....

Weight: ....

Breakfast

_____

_____

_____

_____

_____

Lunch

_____

_____

_____

_____

Water

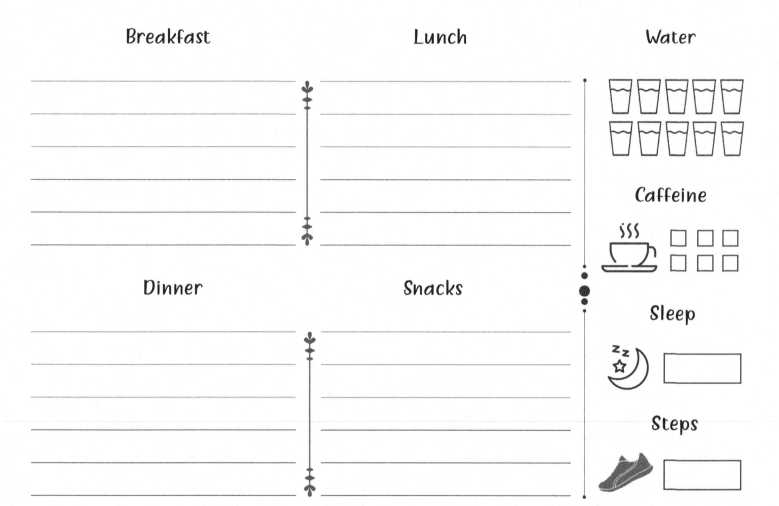

Caffeine

Sleep

Steps

Dinner

_____

_____

_____

_____

Snacks

_____

_____

_____

_____

ACTIVITY/EXERCISE	AMOUNT	NOTES

My Mood is

_____

_____

_____

How to make tomorrow better

_____

_____

_____

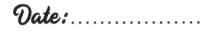

Date: .... Weight: ....

Breakfast

_____
_____
_____
_____
_____

Lunch

_____
_____
_____
_____
_____

Water

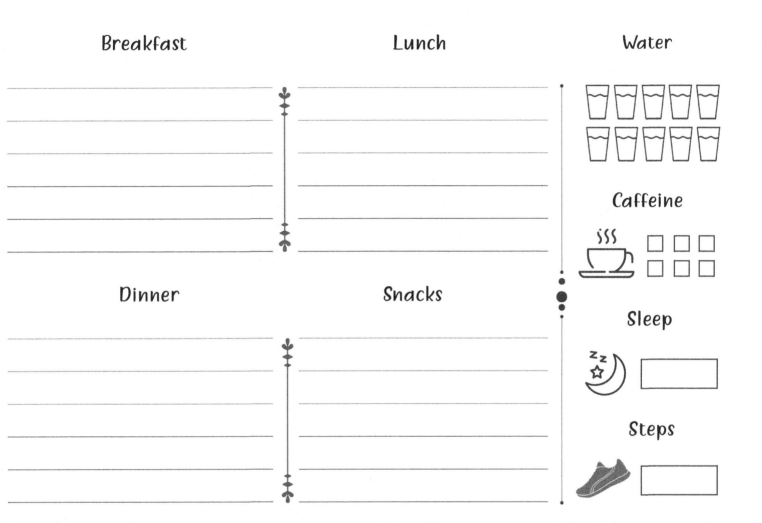

Dinner

_____
_____
_____
_____
_____

Snacks

_____
_____
_____
_____
_____

Caffeine

Sleep

Steps

ACTIVITY/EXERCISE	AMOUNT	NOTES

My Mood is

_____
_____
_____

How to make tomorrow better

_____
_____
_____

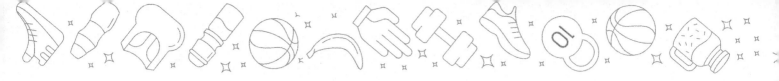

Weekly Check-in

Weekly Goals

☐ _____
_____

☐ _____
_____

☐ _____
_____

Measurements

CHEST	
WAIST	
HIPS	
THIGH	
CALF	
WEIGHT	

Good Habits to Build

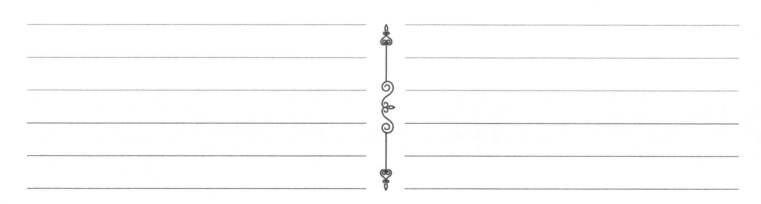

Bad Habits to Cut

How I'm Feeling

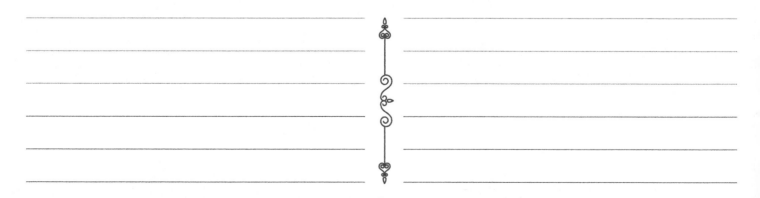

Reasons to keep Going

Date: ....   **Weight:** ....

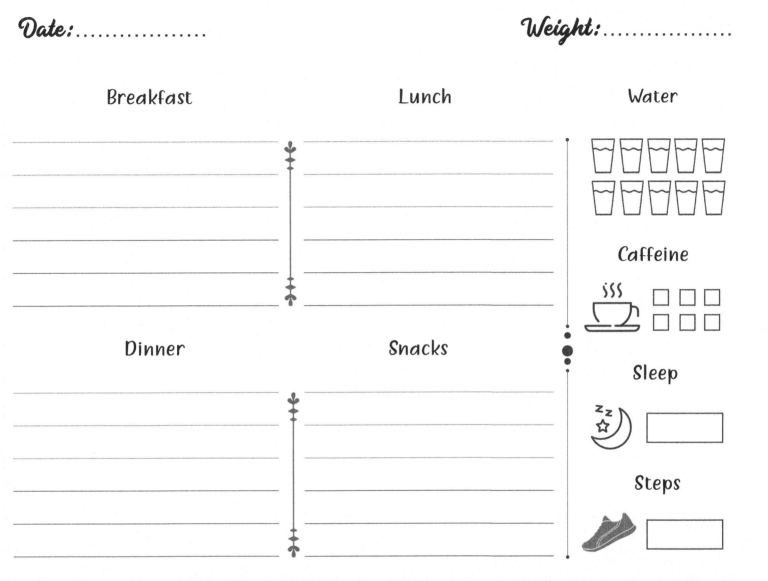

Breakfast

Lunch

Water

Dinner

Snacks

Caffeine

Sleep

Steps

ACTIVITY/EXERCISE	AMOUNT	NOTES

My Mood is

How to make tomorrow better

Date: .... **Weight:** ....

Breakfast

_____
_____
_____
_____

Lunch

_____
_____
_____
_____

Water

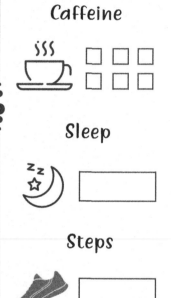

Caffeine

Dinner

_____
_____
_____
_____

Snacks

_____
_____
_____
_____

Sleep

Steps

ACTIVITY/EXERCISE	AMOUNT	NOTES

My Mood is

_____
_____
_____

How to make tomorrow better

_____
_____
_____

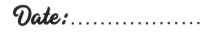

Date: .... **Weight:** ....

Breakfast

_____
_____
_____
_____
_____
_____

Lunch

_____
_____
_____
_____
_____
_____

Water

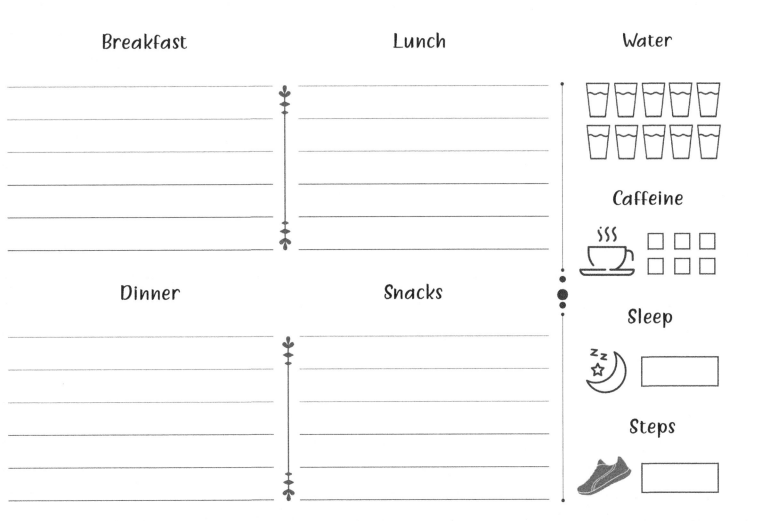

Caffeine

Dinner

_____
_____
_____
_____
_____

Snacks

_____
_____
_____
_____
_____

Sleep

Steps

ACTIVITY/EXERCISE	AMOUNT	NOTES

My Mood is

_____
_____

How to make tomorrow better

_____
_____

Date:................   Weight:................

Breakfast   Lunch   Water

_____   _____
_____   _____
_____   _____   Caffeine
_____   _____
_____   _____
_____   _____

Dinner   Snacks   Sleep

_____   _____
_____   _____
_____   _____   Steps
_____   _____
_____   _____

ACTIVITY/EXERCISE	AMOUNT	NOTES	

My Mood is   How to make tomorrow better

_____   _____
_____   _____
_____   _____

Date: .... Weight: ....

Breakfast

_____
_____
_____
_____
_____

Lunch

_____
_____
_____
_____
_____

Water

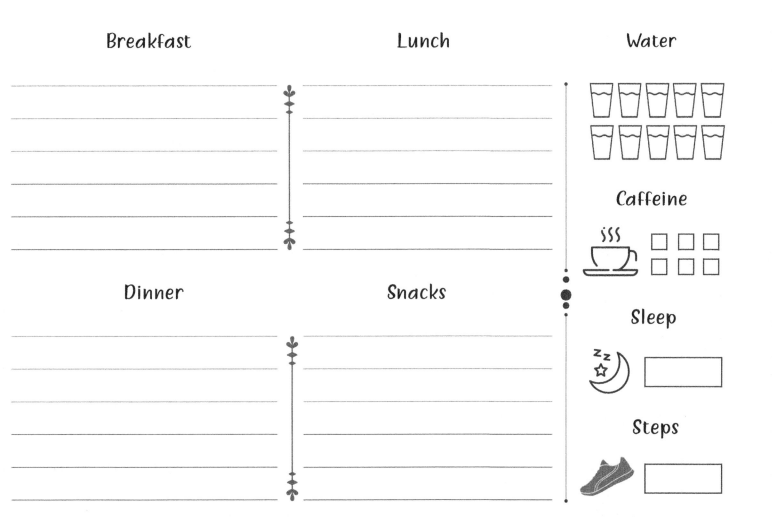

Caffeine

Sleep

Steps

Dinner

_____
_____
_____
_____
_____

Snacks

_____
_____
_____
_____
_____

ACTIVITY/EXERCISE	AMOUNT	NOTES

My Mood is

_____
_____
_____

How to make tomorrow better

_____
_____
_____

Date: .... Weight: ....

Breakfast

Lunch

Water

Dinner

Snacks

Caffeine

Sleep

Steps

ACTIVITY/EXERCISE	AMOUNT	NOTES

My Mood is

How to make tomorrow better

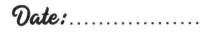

Date: ....   Weight: ....

Breakfast

_____
_____
_____
_____
_____

Lunch

_____
_____
_____
_____
_____

Water

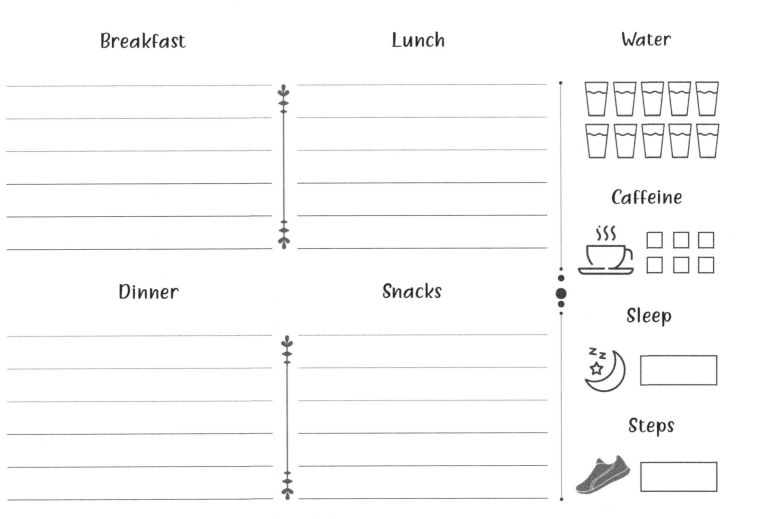

Caffeine

Sleep

Steps

Dinner

_____
_____
_____
_____
_____

Snacks

_____
_____
_____
_____
_____

ACTIVITY/EXERCISE	AMOUNT	NOTES

My Mood is

_____
_____
_____

How to make tomorrow better

_____
_____
_____

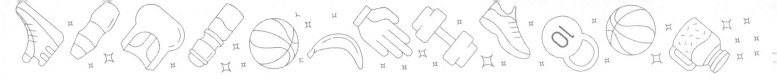

Weekly Check-in

Weekly Goals

☐ _____
_____

☐ _____
_____

☐ _____
_____

Measurements

CHEST	
WAIST	
HIPS	
THIGH	
CALF	
WEIGHT	

Good Habits to Build

_____
_____
_____
_____
_____

Bad Habits to Cut

_____
_____
_____
_____
_____

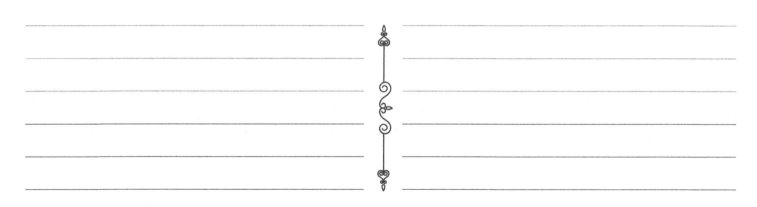

How I'm Feeling

_____
_____
_____
_____

Reasons to keep Going

_____
_____
_____
_____

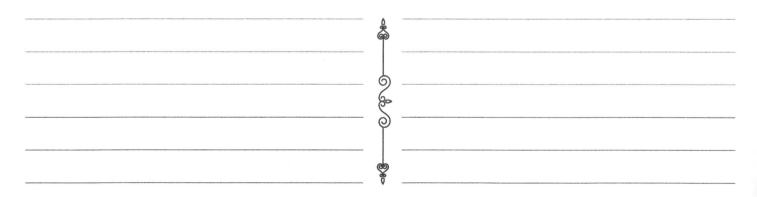

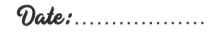 Date:..............

Weight:..............

Breakfast

_____
_____
_____
_____
_____

Lunch

_____
_____
_____
_____
_____

Water

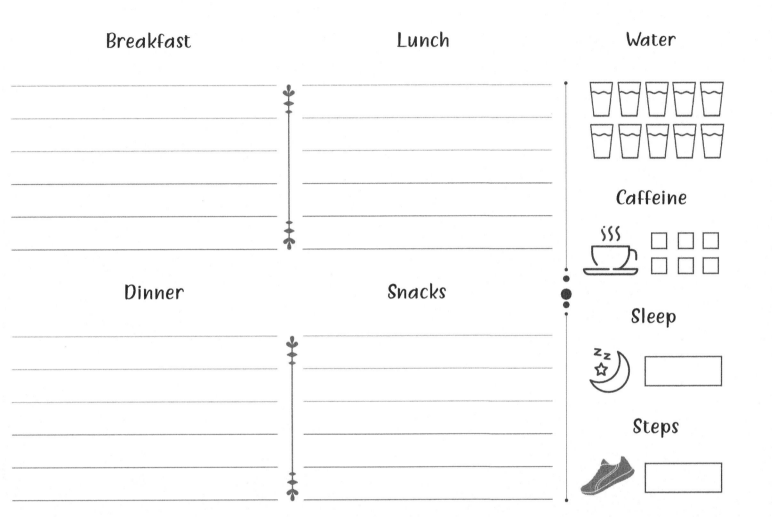

Caffeine

Sleep

Steps

Dinner

_____
_____
_____
_____
_____

Snacks

_____
_____
_____
_____
_____

ACTIVITY/EXERCISE	AMOUNT	NOTES

My Mood is

_____
_____
_____

How to make tomorrow better

_____
_____
_____

Date:................... Weight:...................

Breakfast | Lunch | Water

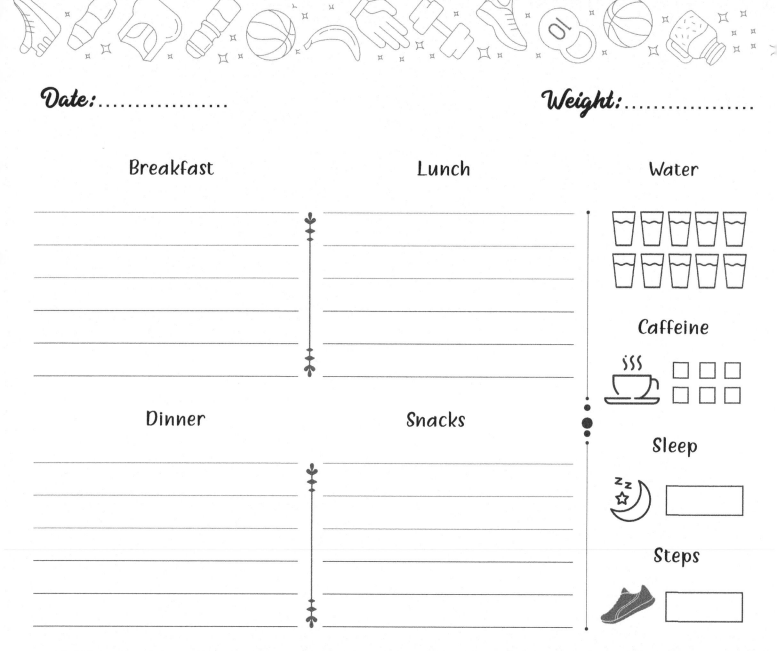

Dinner | Snacks

Caffeine

Sleep

Steps

ACTIVITY/EXERCISE	AMOUNT	NOTES

My Mood is | How to make tomorrow better

Date: ....　　　　　**Weight:** ....

Breakfast

_____
_____
_____
_____
_____
_____

Lunch

_____
_____
_____
_____
_____
_____

Water

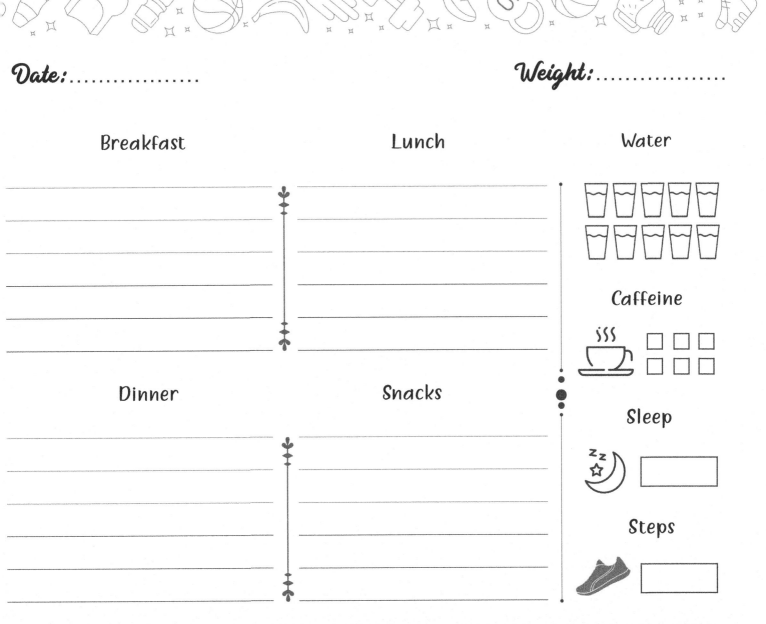

Caffeine

Sleep

Steps

Dinner

_____
_____
_____
_____
_____

Snacks

_____
_____
_____
_____
_____

ACTIVITY/EXERCISE	AMOUNT	NOTES

My Mood is

_____
_____
_____

How to make tomorrow better

_____
_____
_____

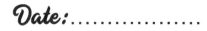 Date:................

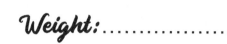 Weight:................

Breakfast

Lunch

Water

Dinner

Snacks

Caffeine

Sleep

Steps

ACTIVITY/EXERCISE	AMOUNT	NOTES

My Mood is

How to make tomorrow better

Date: ....   **Weight:** ....

Breakfast

_____
_____
_____
_____
_____

Lunch

_____
_____
_____
_____
_____

Water

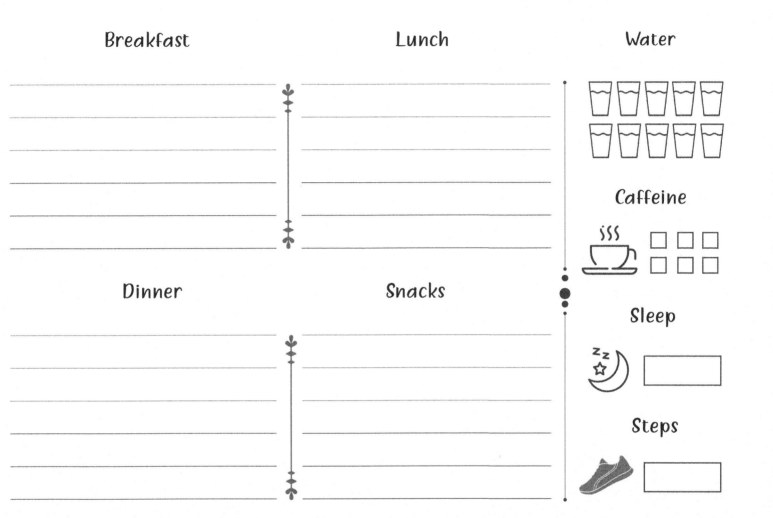

Caffeine

Dinner

_____
_____
_____
_____
_____

Snacks

_____
_____
_____
_____
_____

Sleep

Steps

ACTIVITY/EXERCISE	AMOUNT	NOTES

My Mood is

_____
_____
_____

How to make tomorrow better

_____
_____
_____

Date: ....   **Weight:** ....

Breakfast

_____
_____
_____
_____

Lunch

_____
_____
_____

Water

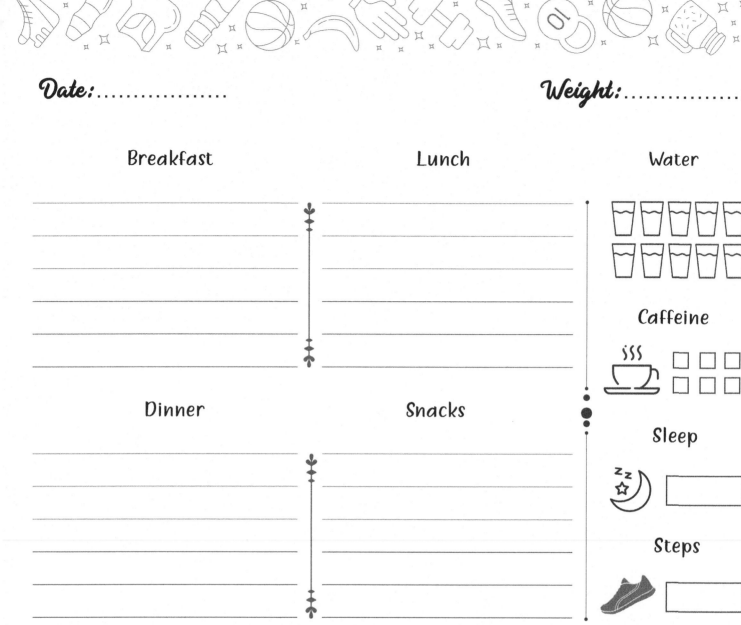

Caffeine

Dinner

_____
_____
_____
_____

Snacks

_____
_____
_____

Sleep

Steps

ACTIVITY/EXERCISE	AMOUNT	NOTES

My Mood is

_____
_____
_____

How to make tomorrow better

_____
_____
_____

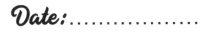

Date: ....

Weight: ....

Breakfast

_____
_____
_____
_____
_____
_____

Lunch

_____
_____
_____
_____
_____
_____

Water

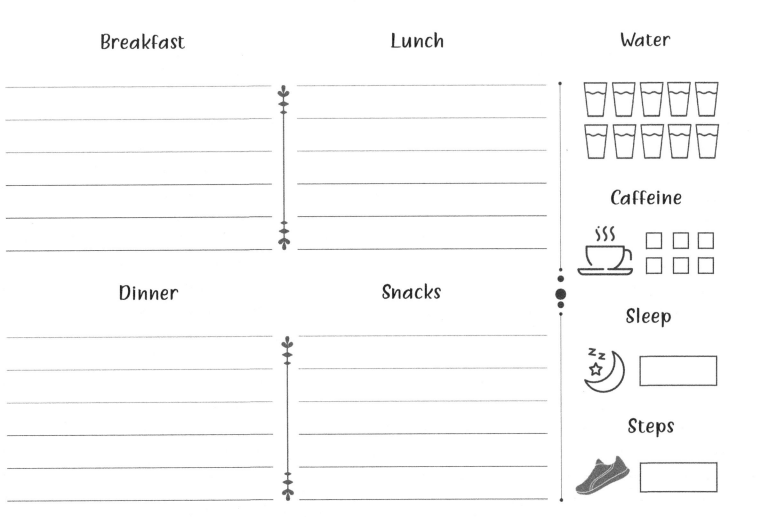

Caffeine

Sleep

Steps

Dinner

_____
_____
_____
_____
_____

Snacks

_____
_____
_____
_____
_____

ACTIVITY/EXERCISE	AMOUNT	NOTES

My Mood is

_____
_____

How to make tomorrow better

_____
_____

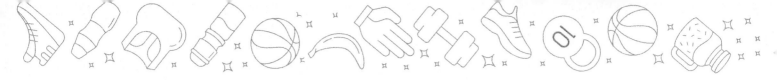

Weekly Check-in

Weekly Goals

☐ _____
_____

☐ _____
_____

☐ _____
_____

Measurements

CHEST	
WAIST	
HIPS	
THIGH	
CALF	
WEIGHT	

Good Habits to Build

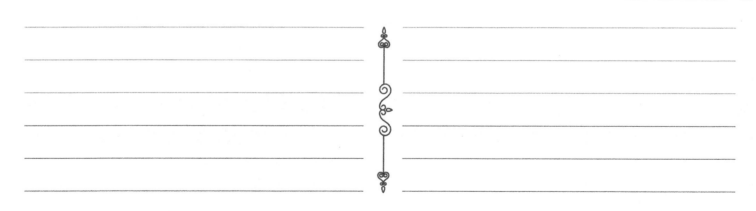

Bad Habits to Cut

How I'm Feeling

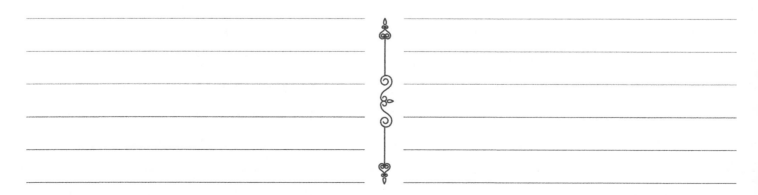

Reasons to keep Going

Date: .... Weight: ....

Breakfast

Lunch

Water

Dinner

Snacks

Caffeine

Sleep

Steps

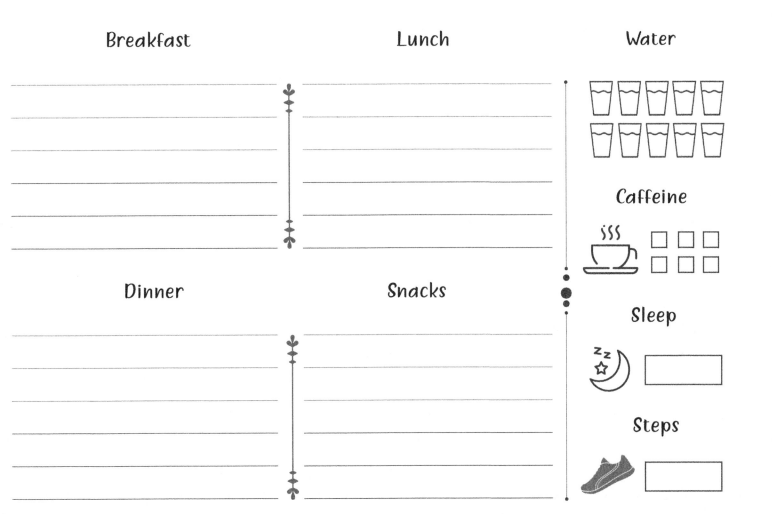

ACTIVITY/EXERCISE	AMOUNT	NOTES

My Mood is

How to make tomorrow better

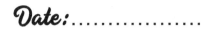

Date: .... **Weight:** ....

Breakfast

_____
_____
_____
_____

Lunch

_____
_____
_____
_____

Water

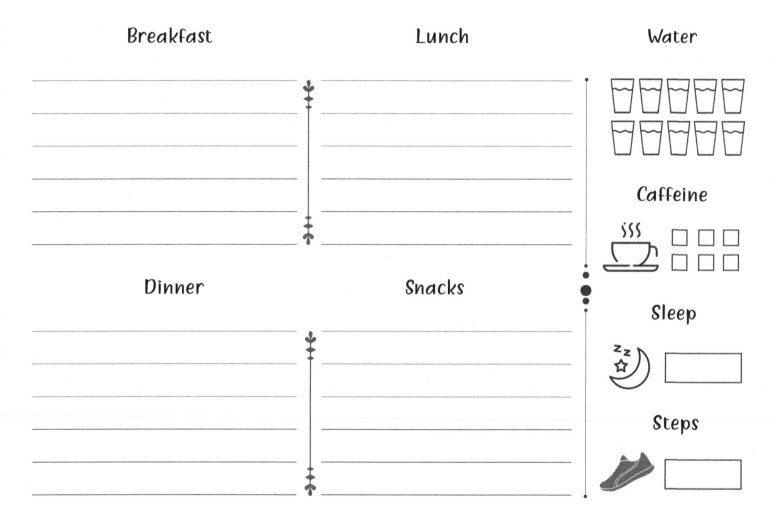

Dinner

_____
_____
_____
_____

Snacks

_____
_____
_____
_____

Caffeine

Sleep

Steps

ACTIVITY/EXERCISE	AMOUNT	NOTES

My Mood is

_____
_____
_____

How to make tomorrow better

_____
_____
_____

Date: ....   Weight: ....

Breakfast

_____
_____
_____
_____
_____
_____

Lunch

_____
_____
_____
_____
_____
_____

Water

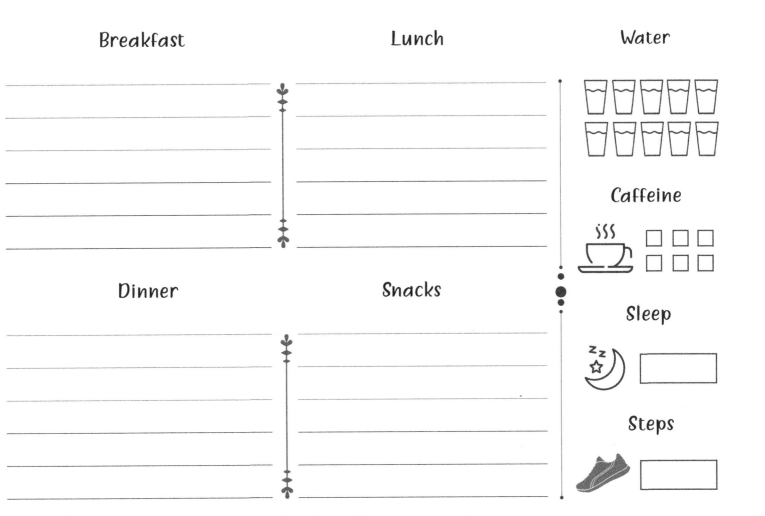

Caffeine

Sleep

Steps

Dinner

_____
_____
_____
_____
_____

Snacks

_____
_____
_____
_____
_____

ACTIVITY/EXERCISE	AMOUNT	NOTES

My Mood is

_____
_____
_____

How to make tomorrow better

_____
_____
_____

Date:................... Weight:...................

Breakfast

Lunch

Water

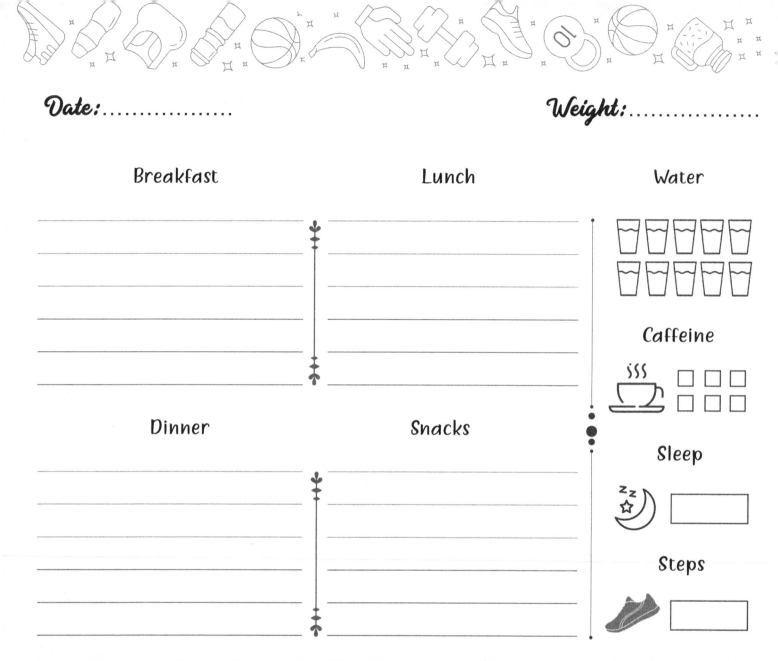

Caffeine

Dinner

Snacks

Sleep

Steps

ACTIVITY/EXERCISE	AMOUNT	NOTES

My Mood is

How to make tomorrow better

Date: ....   Weight: ....

Breakfast   Lunch   Water

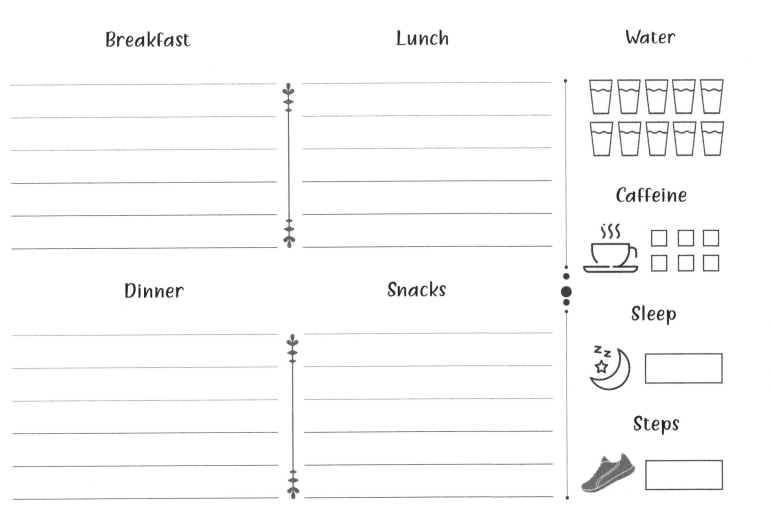

Dinner   Snacks   Caffeine

                                                      Sleep

                                                      Steps

ACTIVITY/EXERCISE	AMOUNT	NOTES

My Mood is   How to make tomorrow better

Date:................... Weight:...................

Breakfast | Lunch | Water

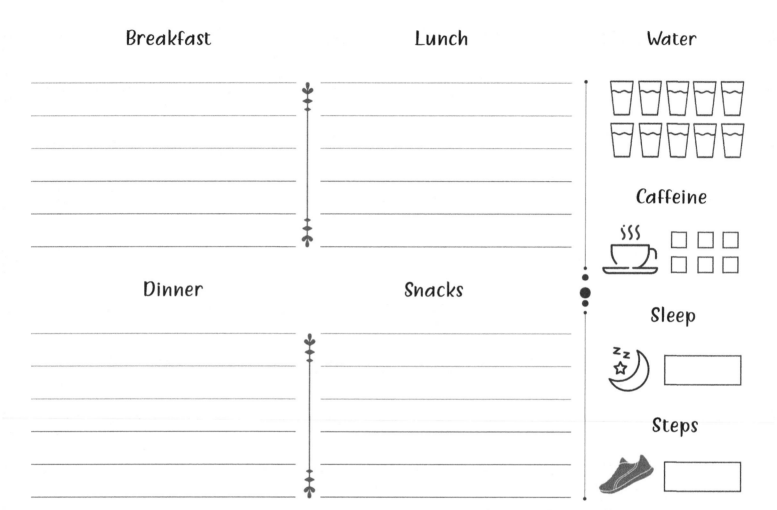

Dinner | Snacks | Caffeine

Sleep

Steps

ACTIVITY/EXERCISE	AMOUNT	NOTES

My Mood is | How to make tomorrow better

Date: ....   **Weight:** ....

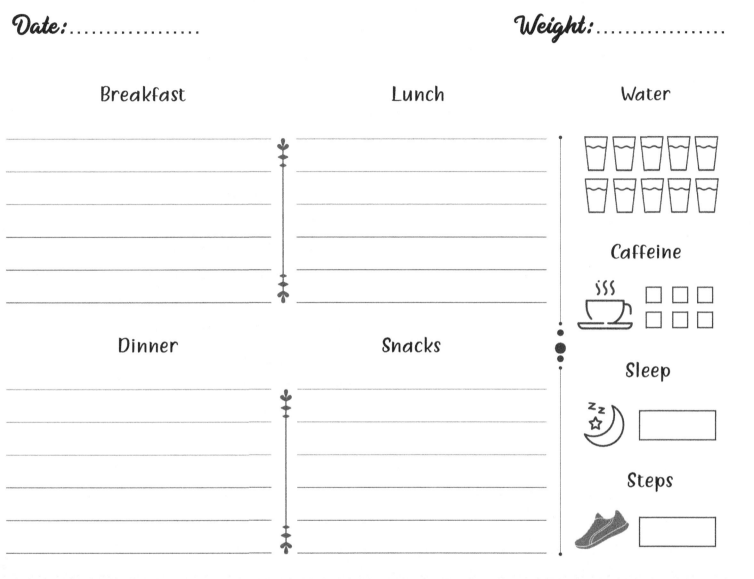

Breakfast	Lunch

Water

Caffeine

Dinner   **Snacks**

Sleep

Steps

ACTIVITY/EXERCISE	AMOUNT	NOTES

My Mood is   How to make tomorrow better

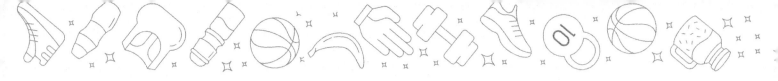

Weekly Check-in

Weekly Goals

☐ _____
_____

☐ _____
_____

☐ _____
_____

Measurements

CHEST	
WAIST	
HIPS	
THIGH	
CALF	
WEIGHT	

Good Habits to Build

_____
_____
_____
_____
_____

Bad Habits to Cut

_____
_____
_____
_____
_____

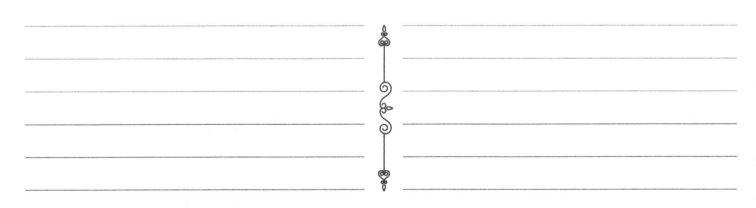

How I'm Feeling

_____
_____
_____
_____

Reasons to keep Going

_____
_____
_____
_____

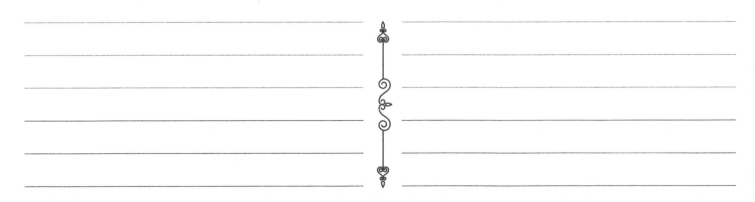

Date:................. Weight:.................

Breakfast

Lunch

Water

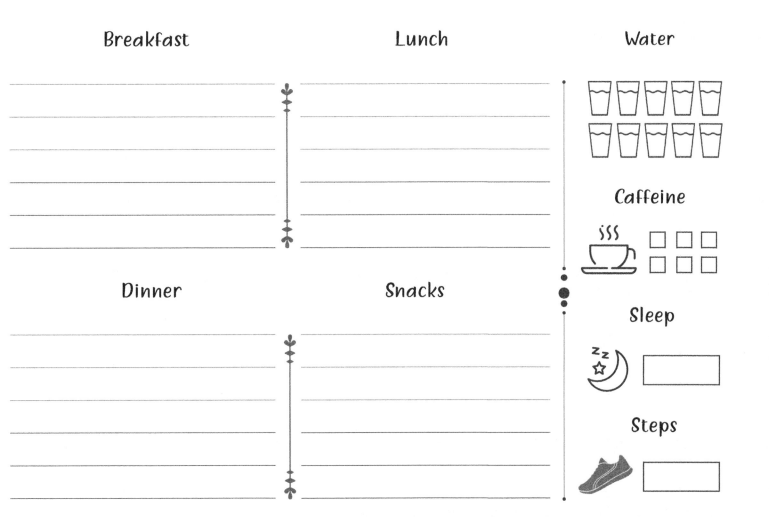

Caffeine

Dinner

Snacks

Sleep

Steps

ACTIVITY/EXERCISE	AMOUNT	NOTES

My Mood is

How to make tomorrow better

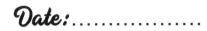

Date: . . . .   **Weight:** . . . .

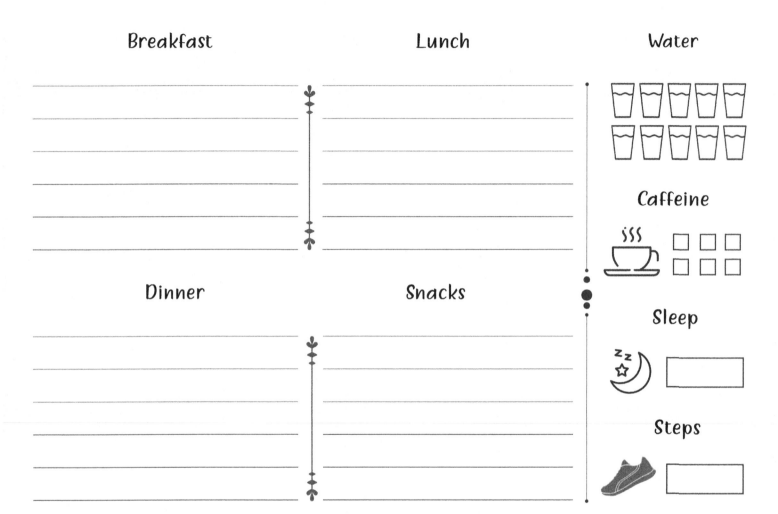

Breakfast

Lunch

Water

Dinner

Snacks

Caffeine

Sleep

Steps

ACTIVITY/EXERCISE	AMOUNT	NOTES	

My Mood is

How to make tomorrow better

Date: .... 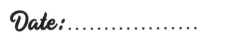 Weight: ....

Breakfast

_____
_____
_____
_____
_____
_____

Lunch

_____
_____
_____
_____
_____
_____

Water

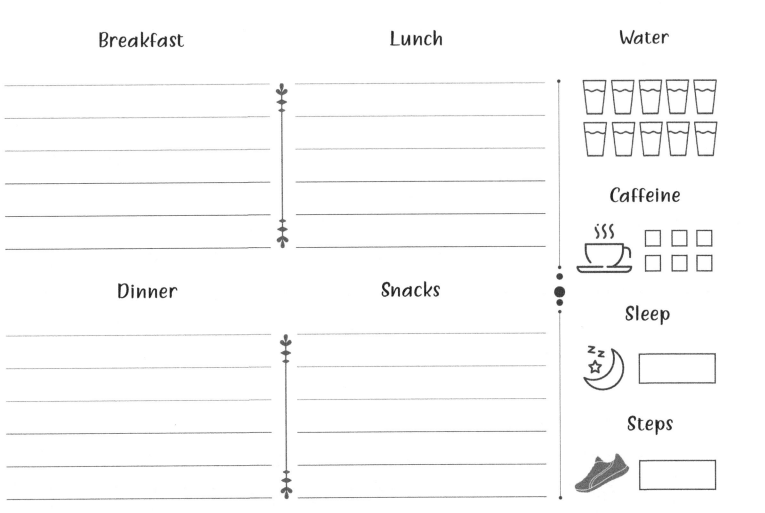

Caffeine

Dinner

_____
_____
_____
_____
_____
_____

Snacks

_____
_____
_____
_____
_____
_____

Sleep

Steps

ACTIVITY/EXERCISE	AMOUNT	NOTES

My Mood is

_____
_____
_____

How to make tomorrow better

_____
_____
_____

Date:........................   **Weight:**....................

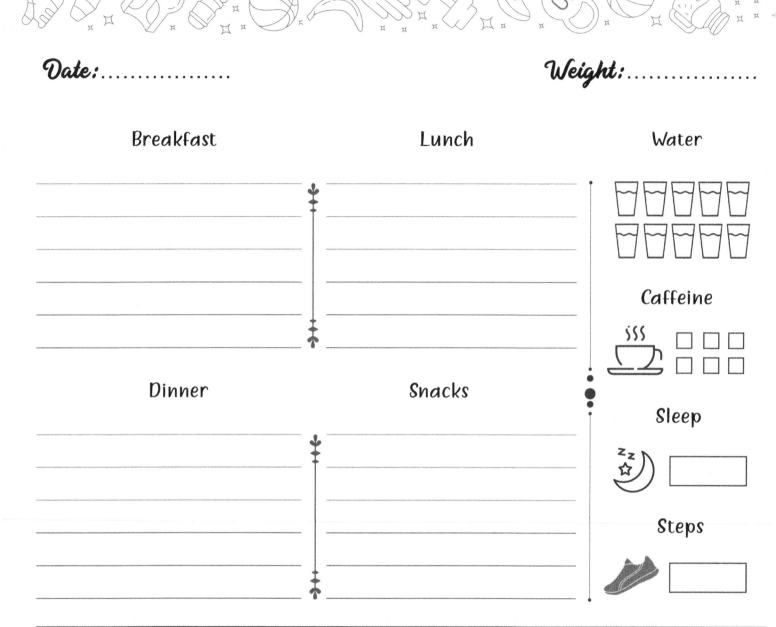

Breakfast	Lunch	Water

Dinner   Snacks

Caffeine

Sleep

Steps

ACTIVITY/EXERCISE	AMOUNT	NOTES

My Mood is   How to make tomorrow better

Date: ....   **Weight:** ....

Breakfast

_____
_____
_____
_____
_____

Lunch

_____
_____
_____
_____
_____

Water

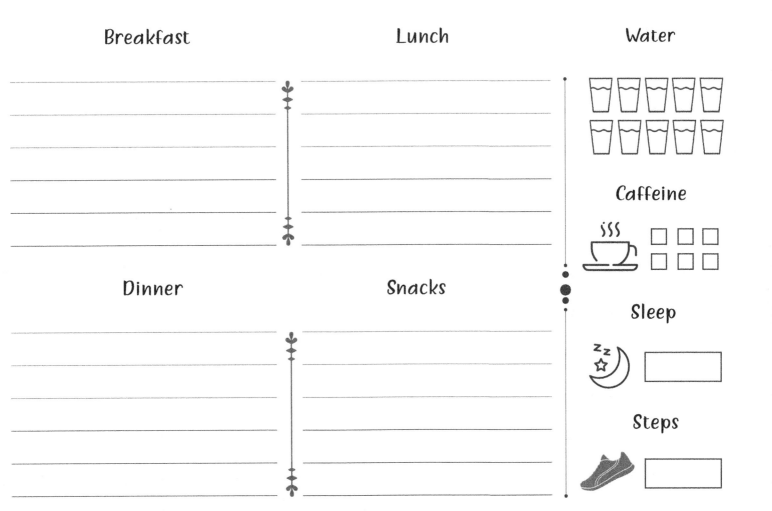

Dinner

_____
_____
_____
_____
_____

Snacks

_____
_____
_____
_____
_____

Caffeine

Sleep

Steps

ACTIVITY/EXERCISE	AMOUNT	NOTES

My Mood is

_____
_____

How to make tomorrow better

_____
_____

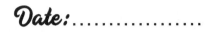

Date: ....   **Weight:** ....

Breakfast   Lunch   Water

Dinner   Snacks

Caffeine

Sleep

Steps

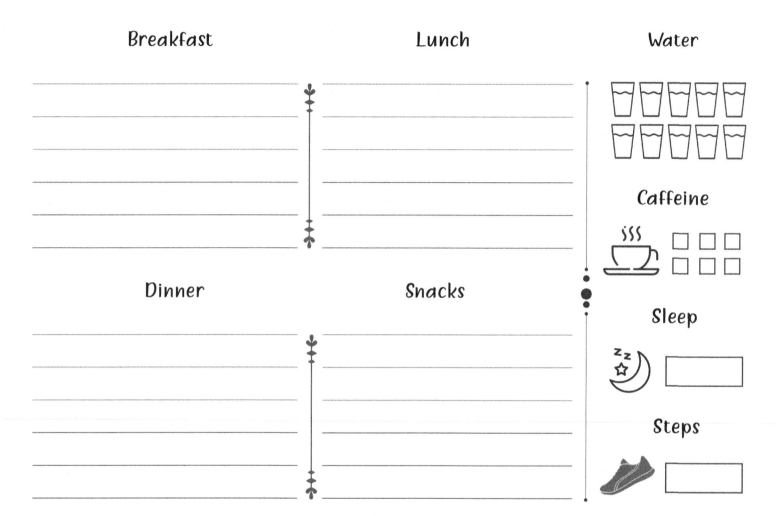

ACTIVITY/EXERCISE	AMOUNT	NOTES

My Mood is   How to make tomorrow better

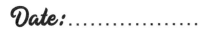

Date: .... **Weight:** ....

Breakfast	Lunch	Water

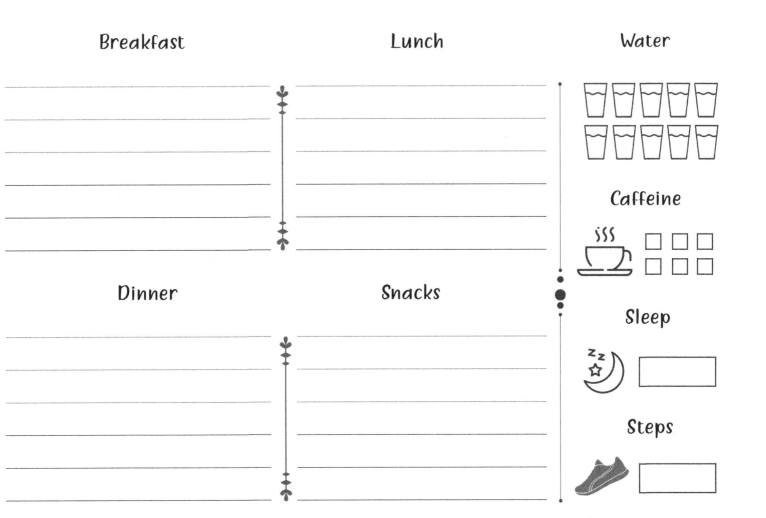

Breakfast
_____
_____
_____
_____
_____
_____

Lunch
_____
_____
_____
_____
_____

Water

Caffeine

Dinner
_____
_____
_____
_____

Snacks
_____
_____
_____
_____

Sleep

Steps

ACTIVITY/EXERCISE	AMOUNT	NOTES

My Mood is
_____
_____
_____

How to make tomorrow better
_____
_____
_____

Weekly Check-in

Weekly Goals

☐ _____
_____

☐ _____
_____

☐ _____
_____

Measurements

CHEST	
WAIST	
HIPS	
THIGH	
CALF	
WEIGHT	

Good Habits to Build

_____
_____
_____
_____
_____

Bad Habits to Cut

_____
_____
_____
_____
_____

How I'm Feeling

_____
_____
_____
_____

Reasons to keep Going

_____
_____
_____
_____

Date: ....   **Weight:** ....

Breakfast

_____
_____
_____
_____
_____

Lunch

_____
_____
_____
_____
_____

Water

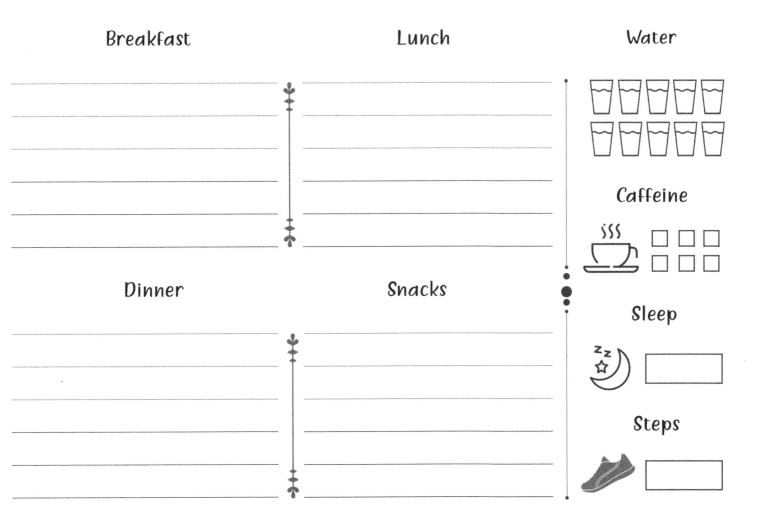

Caffeine

Sleep

Steps

Dinner

_____
_____
_____
_____

Snacks

_____
_____
_____
_____

ACTIVITY/EXERCISE	AMOUNT	NOTES

My Mood is

_____
_____

How to make tomorrow better

_____
_____

Date: ....   **Weight:** ....

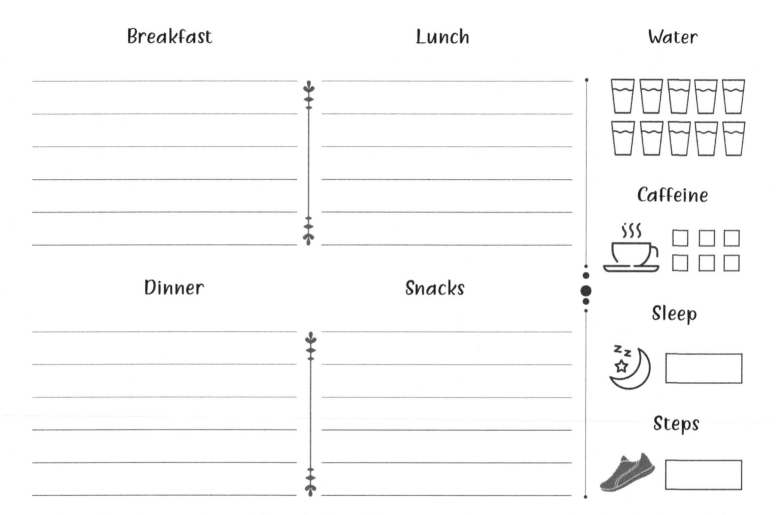

Breakfast

Lunch

Water

Dinner

Snacks

Caffeine

Sleep

Steps

ACTIVITY/EXERCISE	AMOUNT	NOTES

My Mood is

How to make tomorrow better

Date:................ Weight:................

Breakfast

Lunch

Water

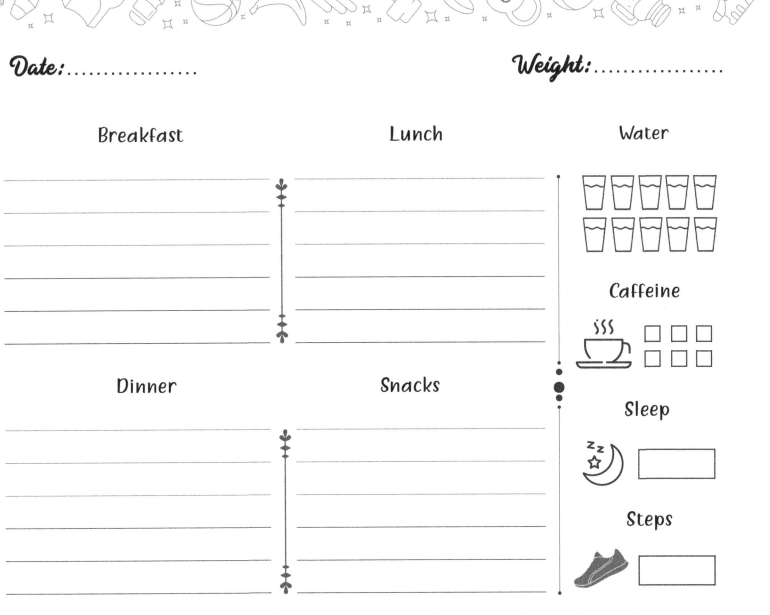

Caffeine

Dinner

Snacks

Sleep

Steps

ACTIVITY/EXERCISE	AMOUNT	NOTES

My Mood is

How to make tomorrow better

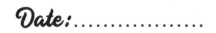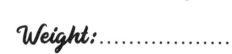

Date: ....   **Weight:** ....

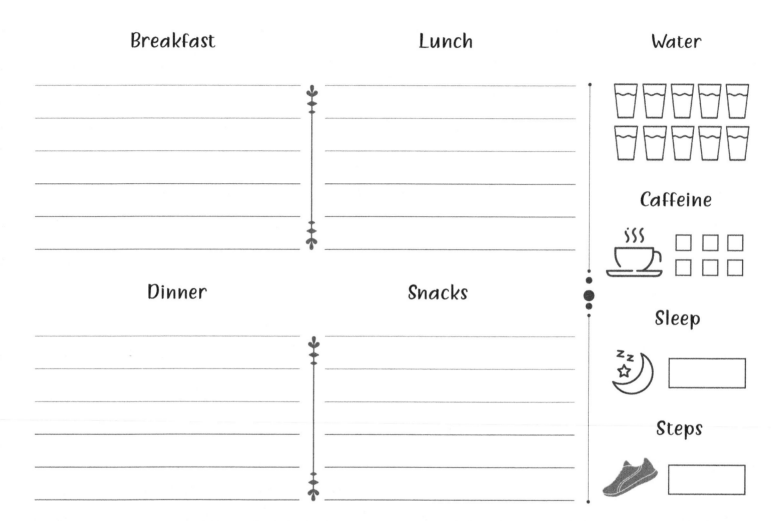

Breakfast	Lunch	Water

Caffeine

Dinner   Snacks

Sleep

Steps

ACTIVITY/EXERCISE	AMOUNT	NOTES	

My Mood is   How to make tomorrow better

Date: .... Weight: ....

Breakfast	Lunch	Water

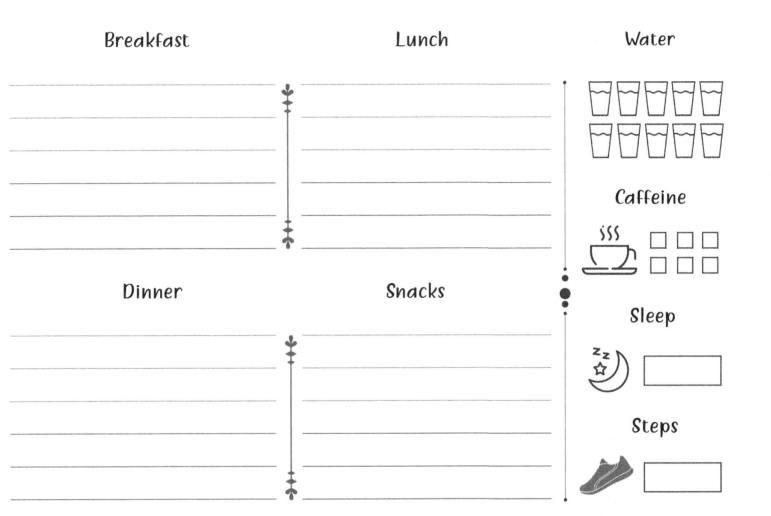

Caffeine

Dinner

Snacks

Sleep

Steps

ACTIVITY/EXERCISE	AMOUNT	NOTES

My Mood is

How to make tomorrow better

Date: ....   Weight: ....

Breakfast   Lunch   Water

_____   _____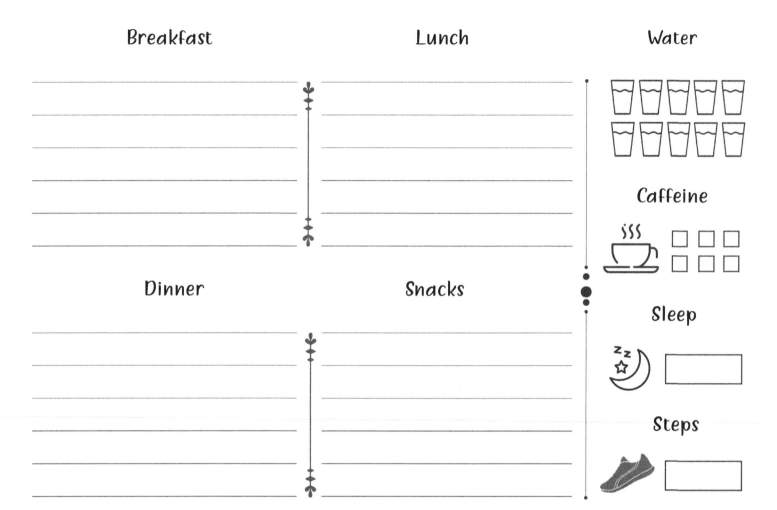
_____   _____
_____   _____
_____   _____
_____   _____

                                                  Caffeine

Dinner   Snacks

_____   _____   Sleep
_____   _____
_____   _____
_____   _____   Steps
_____   _____

ACTIVITY/EXERCISE	AMOUNT	NOTES

My Mood is   How to make tomorrow better

_____   _____
_____   _____
_____   _____

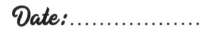

Date: ....   **Weight:** ....

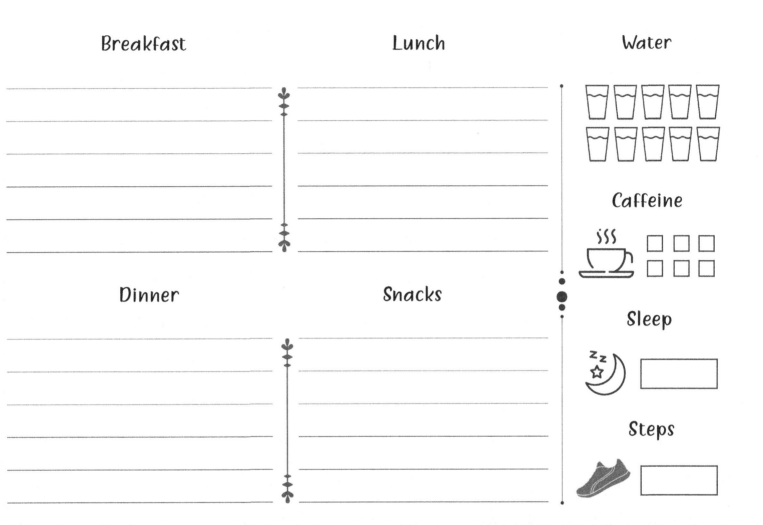

Breakfast	Lunch	Water

Caffeine

Dinner   Snacks

Sleep

Steps

ACTIVITY/EXERCISE	AMOUNT	NOTES

My Mood is   How to make tomorrow better

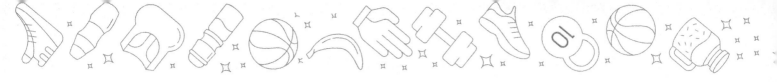

Weekly Check-in

Weekly Goals

☐ _____
_____

☐ _____
_____

☐ _____
_____

Measurements

CHEST	
WAIST	
HIPS	
THIGH	
CALF	
WEIGHT	

Good Habits to Build

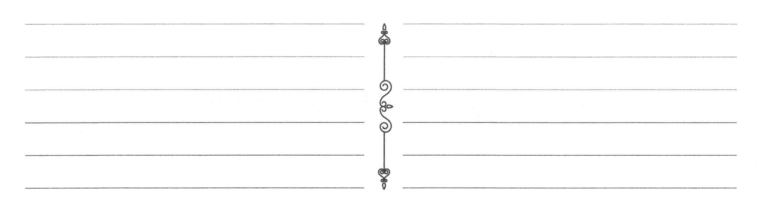

Bad Habits to Cut

How I'm Feeling

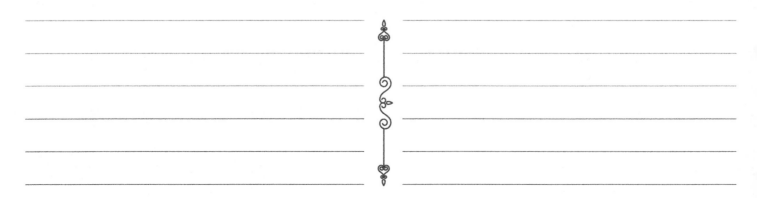

Reasons to keep Going

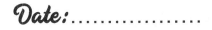

Date:..................   Weight:..................

Breakfast   Lunch   Water

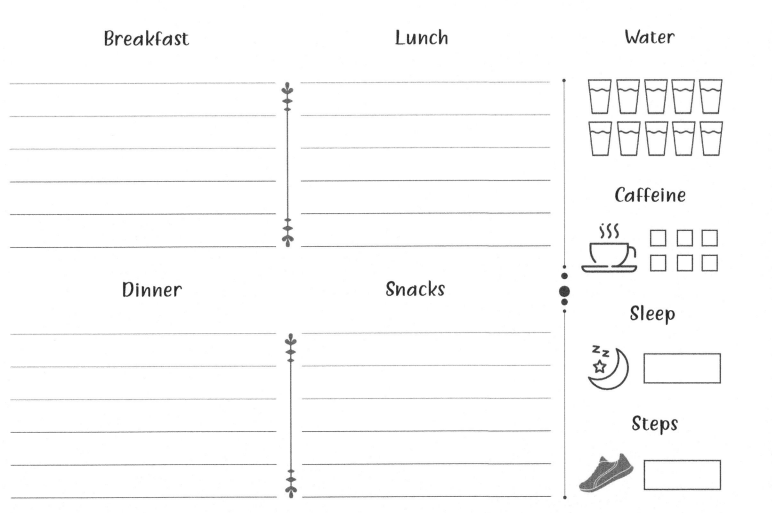

_____   _____
_____   _____
_____   _____
_____   _____

Dinner   Snacks   Caffeine

_____   _____
_____   _____   Sleep
_____   _____
_____   _____   Steps

ACTIVITY/EXERCISE	AMOUNT	NOTES

My Mood is   How to make tomorrow better

_____   _____
_____   _____
_____   _____

Date:.................. Weight:..................

Breakfast

Lunch

Water

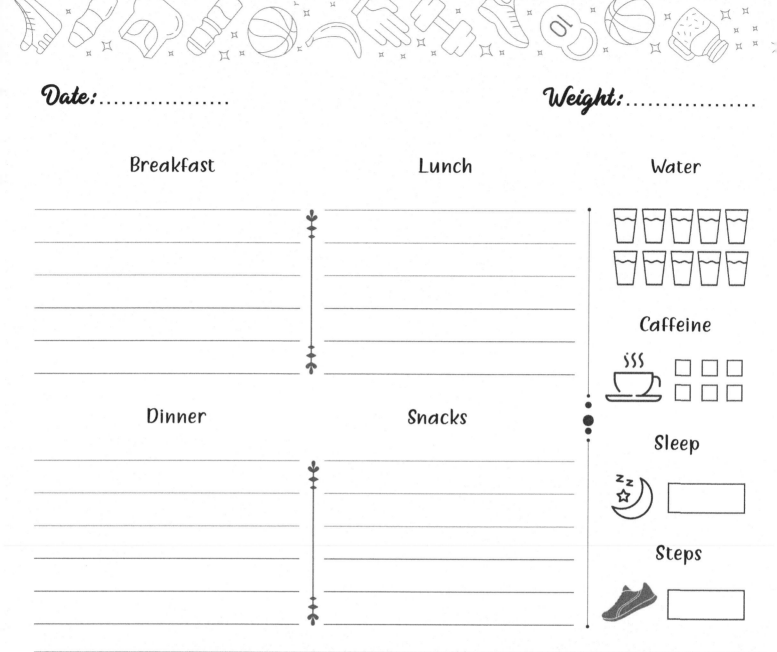

Dinner

Snacks

Caffeine

Sleep

Steps

ACTIVITY/EXERCISE	AMOUNT	NOTES

My Mood is

How to make tomorrow better

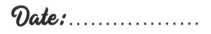

Date: .... Weight: ....

Breakfast

Lunch

Water

Dinner

Snacks

Caffeine

Sleep

Steps

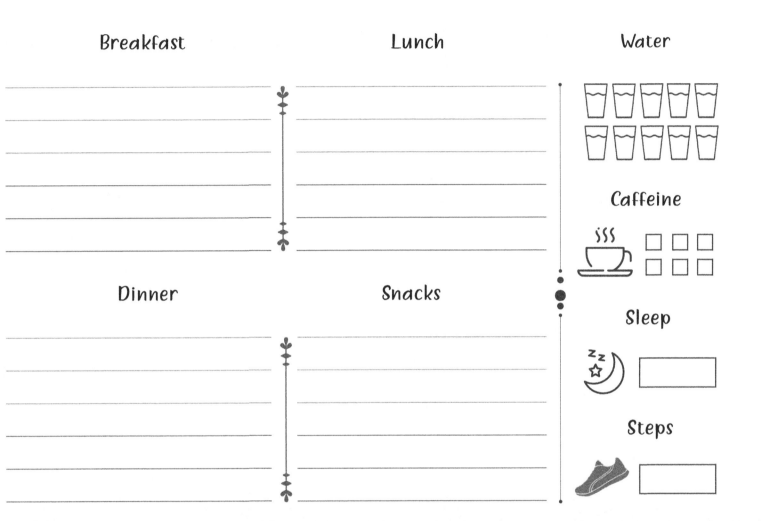

ACTIVITY/EXERCISE	AMOUNT	NOTES

My Mood is

How to make tomorrow better

Date: .... Weight: ....

Breakfast

Lunch

Water

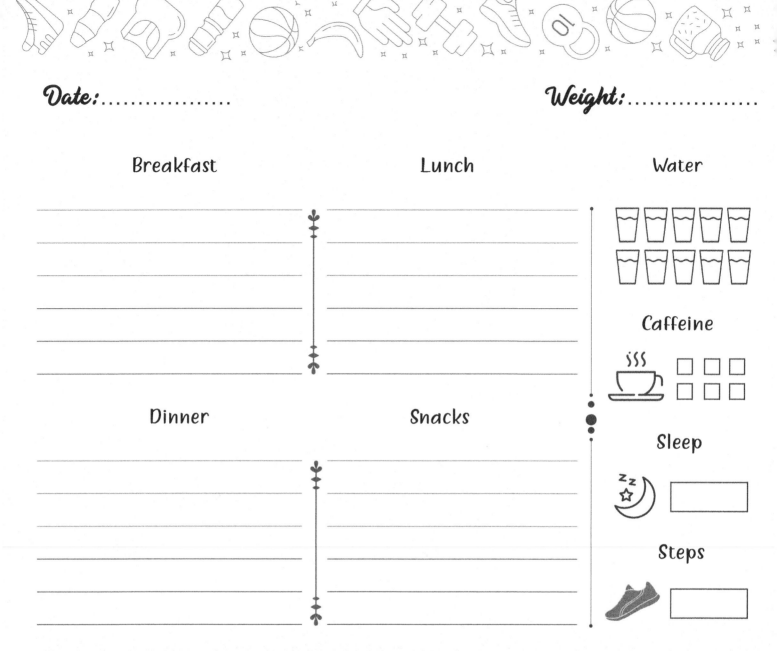

Caffeine

Dinner

Snacks

Sleep

Steps

ACTIVITY/EXERCISE	AMOUNT	NOTES

My Mood is

How to make tomorrow better

Date: .... Weight: ....

Breakfast

Lunch

Water

Dinner

Snacks

Caffeine

Sleep

Steps

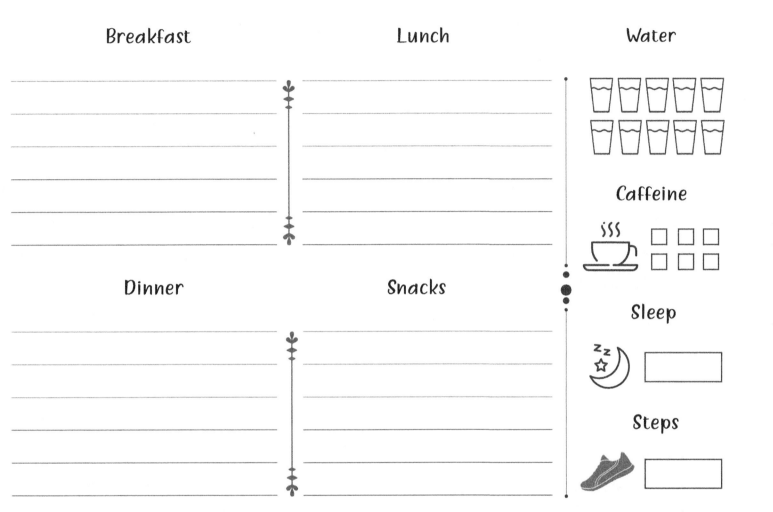

ACTIVITY/EXERCISE	AMOUNT	NOTES

My Mood is

How to make tomorrow better

Date:................   Weight:................

Breakfast   ### Lunch   ### Water

_____   _____
_____   _____
_____   _____
_____   _____
_____   _____

Dinner   ### Snacks   ### Caffeine

_____   _____
_____   _____   ### Sleep
_____   _____
_____   _____   ### Steps
_____   _____

ACTIVITY/EXERCISE	AMOUNT	NOTES

My Mood is   ### How to make tomorrow better

_____   _____
_____   _____
_____   _____

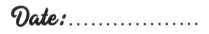

Date: ....   Weight: ....

Breakfast

_____
_____
_____
_____
_____

Lunch

_____
_____
_____
_____
_____

Water

Caffeine

Dinner

_____
_____
_____
_____

Snacks

_____
_____
_____
_____
_____

Sleep

Steps

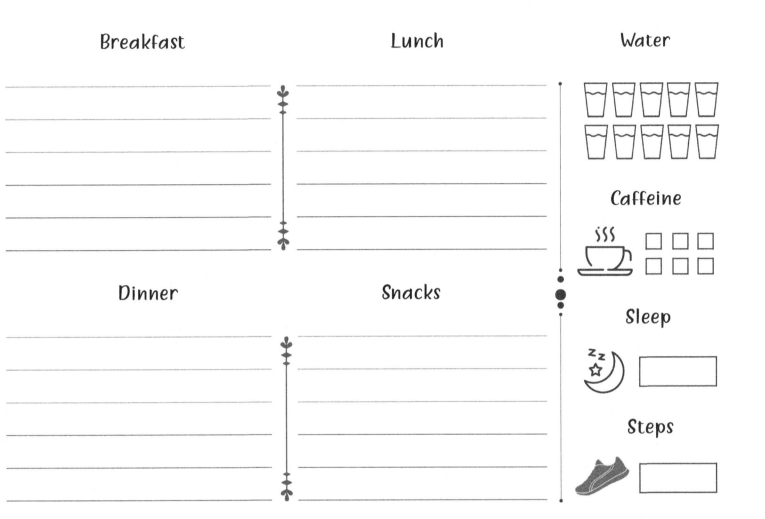

ACTIVITY/EXERCISE	AMOUNT	NOTES

My Mood is

_____
_____
_____

How to make tomorrow better

_____
_____
_____

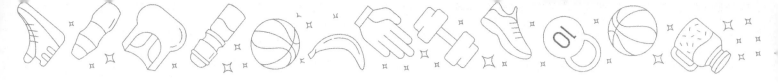

Weekly Check-in

Weekly Goals

☐ _____
_____

☐ _____
_____

☐ _____
_____

Measurements

CHEST	
WAIST	
HIPS	
THIGH	
CALF	
WEIGHT	

Good Habits to Build

_____
_____
_____
_____
_____

Bad Habits to Cut

_____
_____
_____
_____
_____

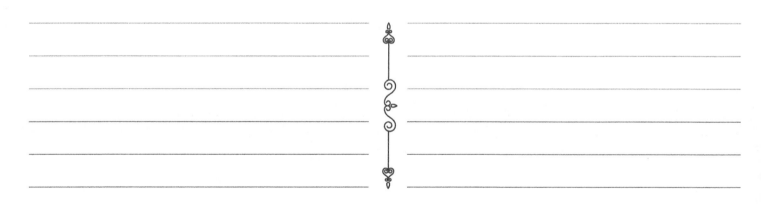

How I'm Feeling

_____
_____
_____
_____

Reasons to keep Going

_____
_____
_____
_____

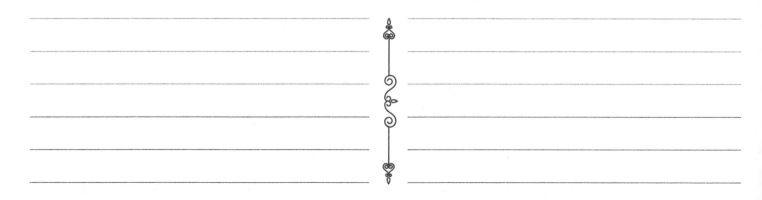

Date: .... Weight: ....

Breakfast

Lunch

Water

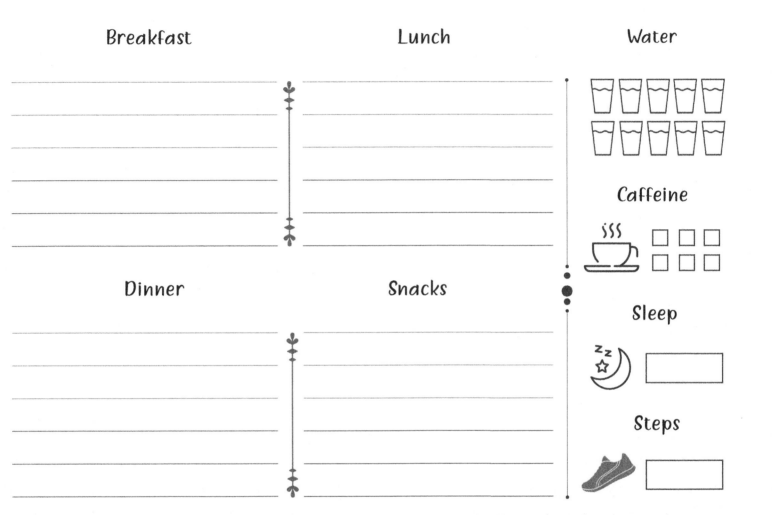

Caffeine

Dinner

Snacks

Sleep

Steps

ACTIVITY/EXERCISE	AMOUNT	NOTES

My Mood is

How to make tomorrow better

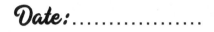

Date: .... Weight: ....

Breakfast

_____
_____
_____
_____
_____

Lunch

_____
_____
_____
_____
_____

Water

Caffeine

Sleep

Steps

Dinner

_____
_____
_____
_____
_____

Snacks

_____
_____
_____
_____
_____

ACTIVITY/EXERCISE	AMOUNT	NOTES

My Mood is

_____
_____
_____

How to make tomorrow better

_____
_____
_____

Date: .... Weight: ....

Breakfast

Lunch

Water

Dinner

Snacks

Caffeine

Sleep

Steps

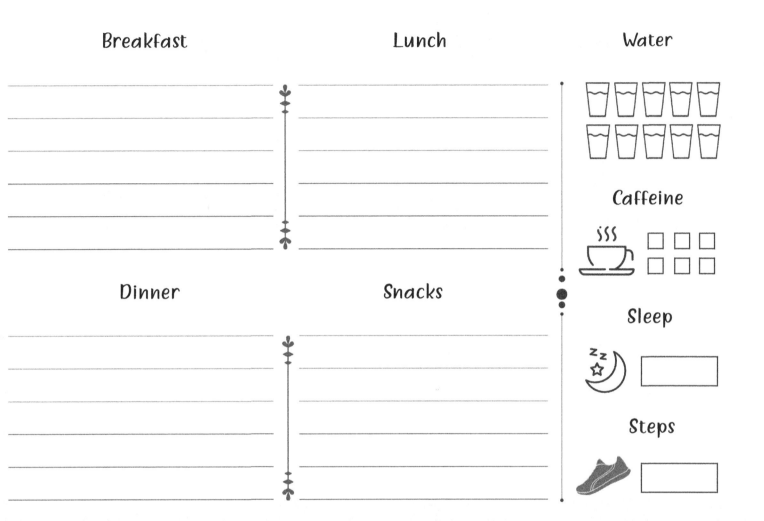

ACTIVITY/EXERCISE	AMOUNT	NOTES

My Mood is

How to make tomorrow better

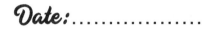

Date: ....   **Weight:** ....

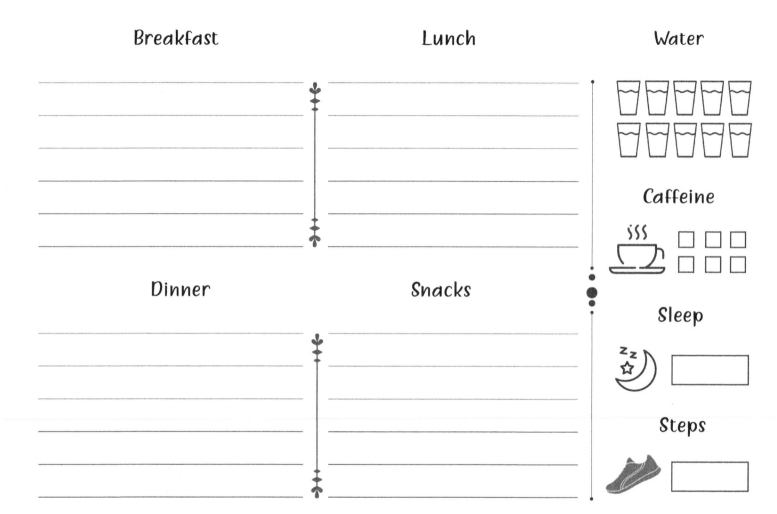

Breakfast
_____
_____
_____
_____
_____
_____

Lunch
_____
_____
_____
_____
_____
_____

Water

Caffeine

Sleep

Steps

Dinner
_____
_____
_____
_____
_____
_____

Snacks
_____
_____
_____
_____
_____
_____

ACTIVITY/EXERCISE	AMOUNT	NOTES

My Mood is
_____
_____

How to make tomorrow better
_____
_____
_____

Date:................. Weight:.................

Breakfast

_____
_____
_____
_____
_____

Lunch

_____
_____
_____
_____
_____

Water

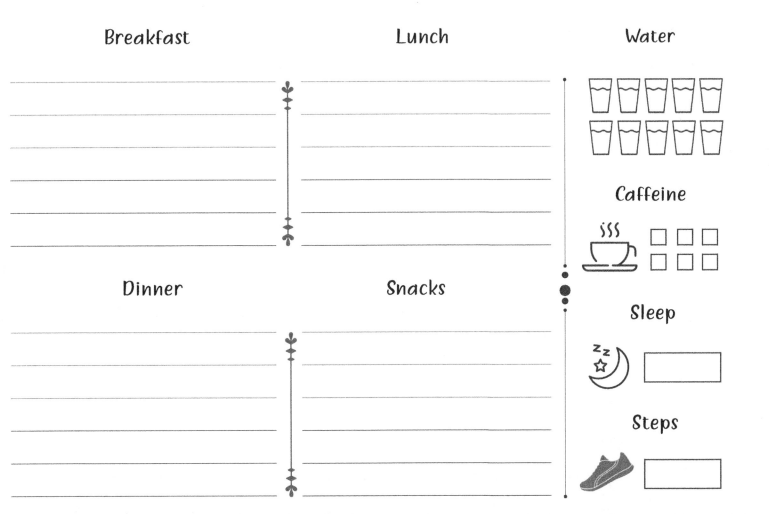

Dinner

_____
_____
_____
_____
_____

Snacks

_____
_____
_____
_____
_____

Caffeine

Sleep

Steps

ACTIVITY/EXERCISE	AMOUNT	NOTES

My Mood is

_____
_____

How to make tomorrow better

_____
_____

Date:................   Weight:................

Breakfast   Lunch   Water

_____   _____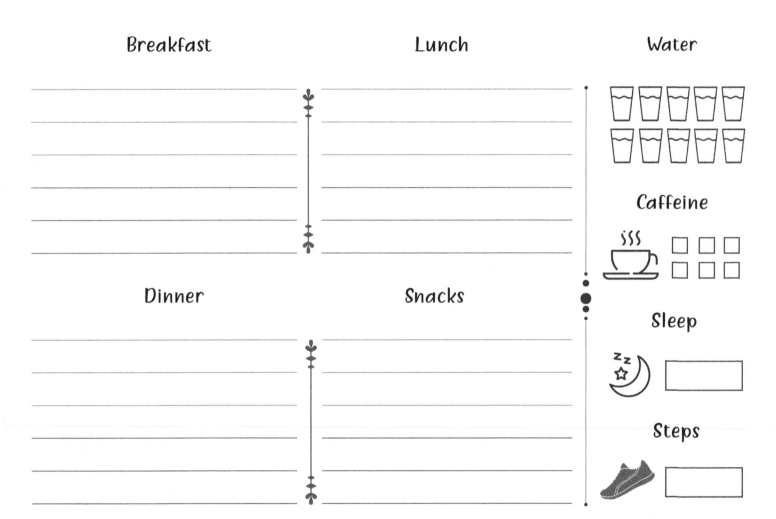

_____   _____

_____   _____

_____   _____   Caffeine

_____   _____

Dinner   Snacks

_____   _____   Sleep

_____   _____

_____   _____

_____   _____   Steps

_____   _____

ACTIVITY/EXERCISE	AMOUNT	NOTES

My Mood is   How to make tomorrow better

_____   _____

_____   _____

_____   _____

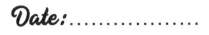

Date: ....

Weight: ....

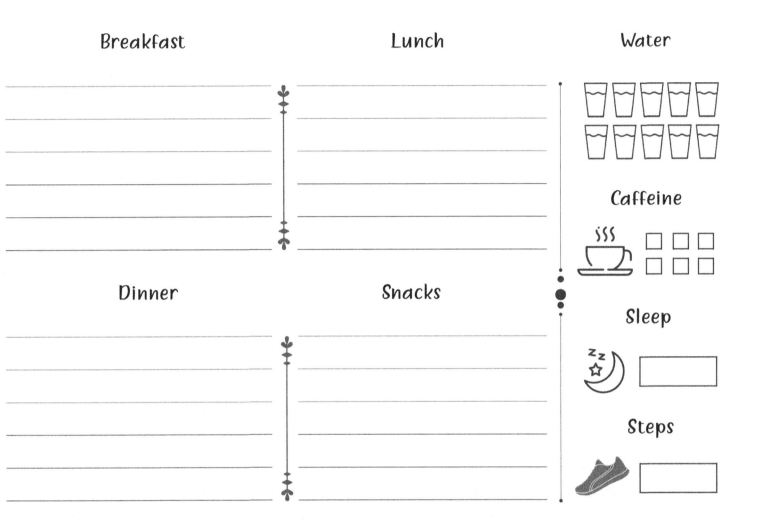

Breakfast

Lunch

Water

Dinner

Snacks

Caffeine

Sleep

Steps

ACTIVITY/EXERCISE	AMOUNT	NOTES

My Mood is

How to make tomorrow better

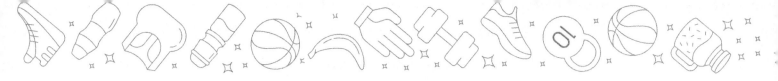

Weekly Check-in

Weekly Goals

☐ _____
_____

☐ _____
_____

☐ _____
_____

Measurements

CHEST	
WAIST	
HIPS	
THIGH	
CALF	
WEIGHT	

Good Habits to Build

_____
_____
_____
_____

Bad Habits to Cut

_____
_____
_____
_____

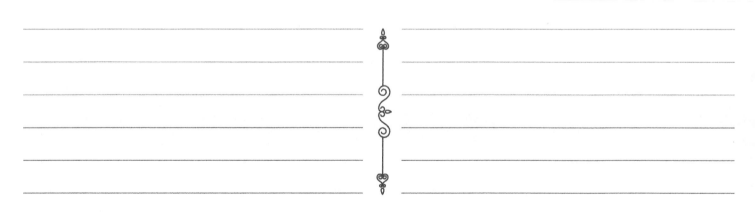

How I'm Feeling

_____
_____
_____
_____

Reasons to keep Going

_____
_____
_____
_____

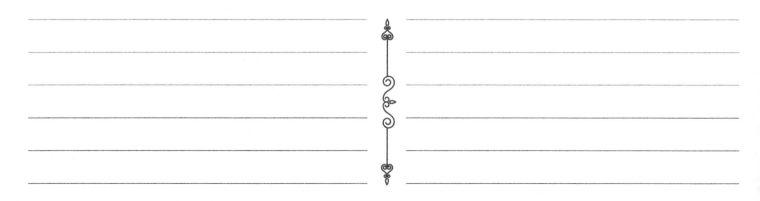

Date: . . . .　　　　　Weight: . . . .

Breakfast　　　　　Lunch　　　　　Water

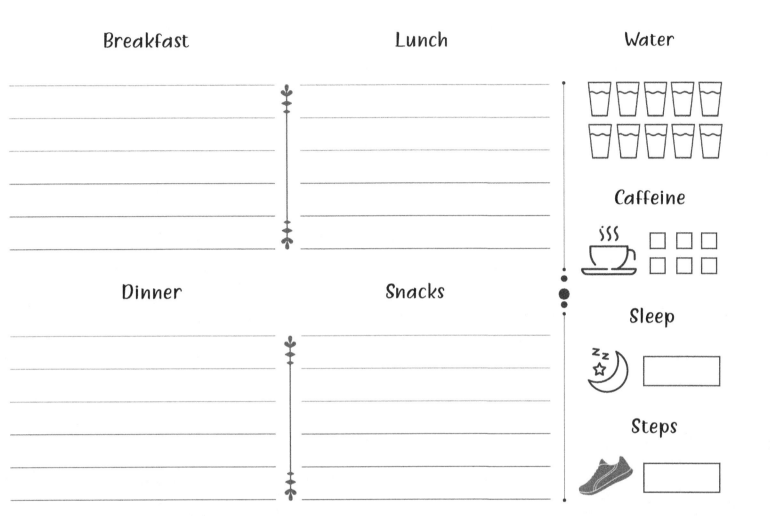

Caffeine

Dinner　　　　　Snacks

Sleep

Steps

ACTIVITY/EXERCISE	AMOUNT	NOTES

My Mood is　　　　　How to make tomorrow better

Date: ....

Weight: ....

Breakfast

_____
_____
_____
_____

Lunch

_____
_____
_____
_____

Water

Caffeine

Dinner

_____
_____
_____
_____

Snacks

_____
_____
_____
_____

Sleep

Steps

ACTIVITY/EXERCISE	AMOUNT	NOTES

My Mood is

_____
_____
_____

How to make tomorrow better

_____
_____
_____

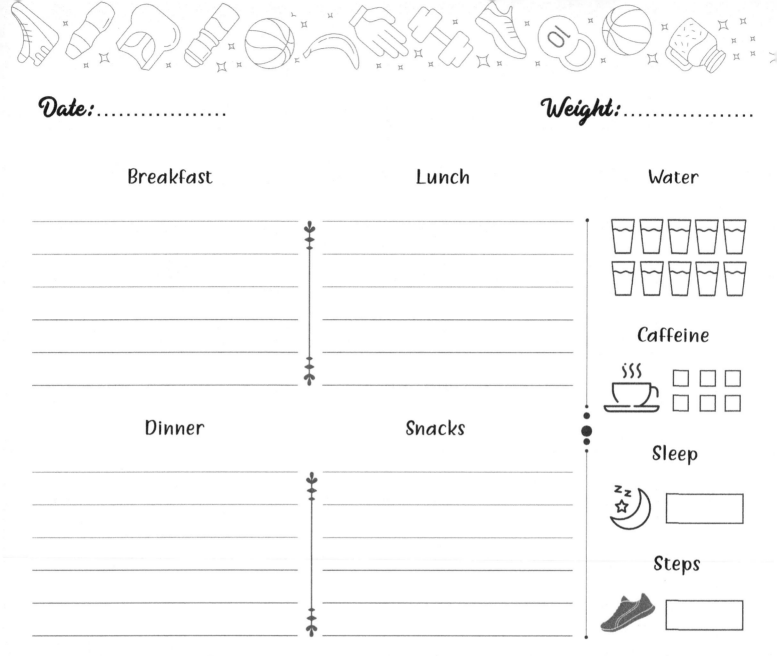

Date: . . . .   Weight: . . . .

Breakfast   Lunch   Water

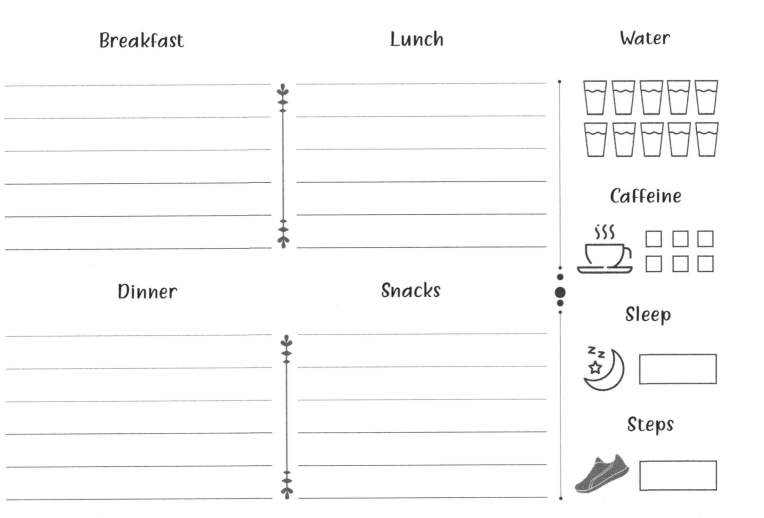

Caffeine

Dinner   Snacks

Sleep

Steps

ACTIVITY/EXERCISE	AMOUNT	NOTES

My Mood is   How to make tomorrow better

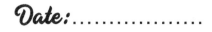

Date: ....   **Weight:** ....

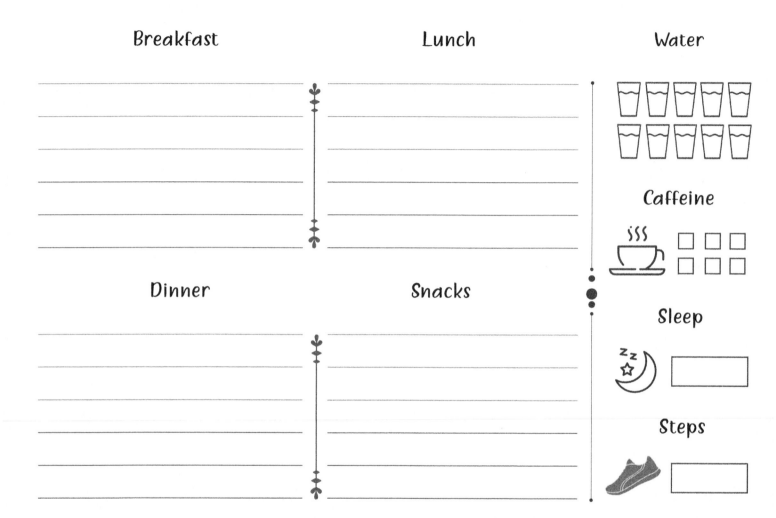

Breakfast
_____
_____
_____
_____
_____

Lunch
_____
_____
_____
_____
_____

Water

Caffeine

Dinner
_____
_____
_____
_____
_____

Snacks
_____
_____
_____
_____
_____

Sleep

Steps

ACTIVITY/EXERCISE	AMOUNT	NOTES	

My Mood is
_____
_____
_____

How to make tomorrow better
_____
_____
_____

Date: ....   **Weight:** ....

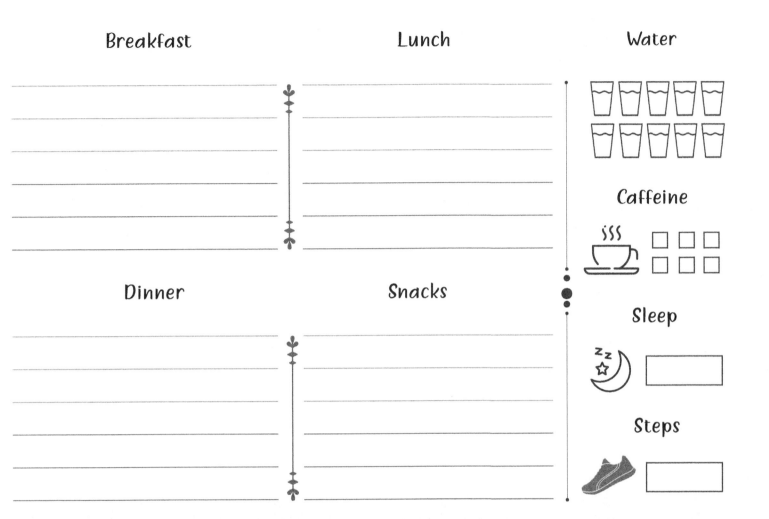

Breakfast	Lunch	Water

Dinner   Snacks

Caffeine

Sleep

Steps

ACTIVITY/EXERCISE	AMOUNT	NOTES

My Mood is   How to make tomorrow better

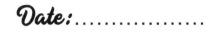

Date: .... Weight: ....

Breakfast

_____
_____
_____
_____
_____

Lunch

_____
_____
_____
_____
_____

Water

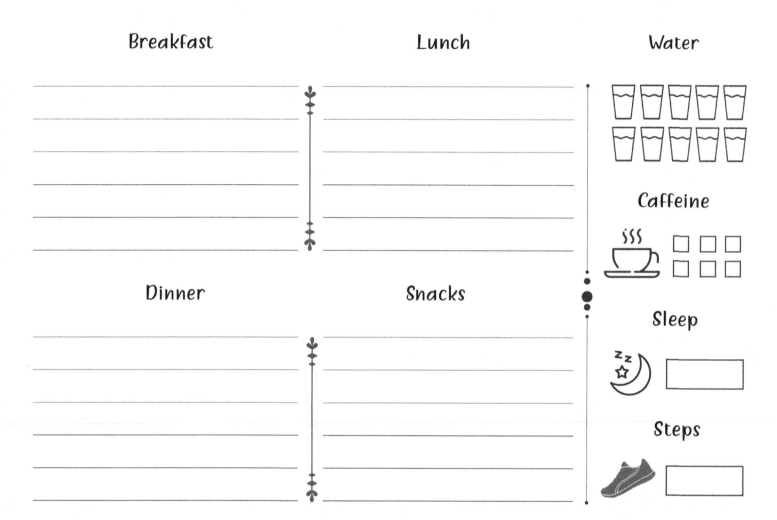

Caffeine

Sleep

Steps

Dinner

_____
_____
_____
_____
_____

Snacks

_____
_____
_____
_____
_____

ACTIVITY/EXERCISE	AMOUNT	NOTES

My Mood is

_____
_____
_____

How to make tomorrow better

_____
_____
_____

Date: ....   Weight: ....

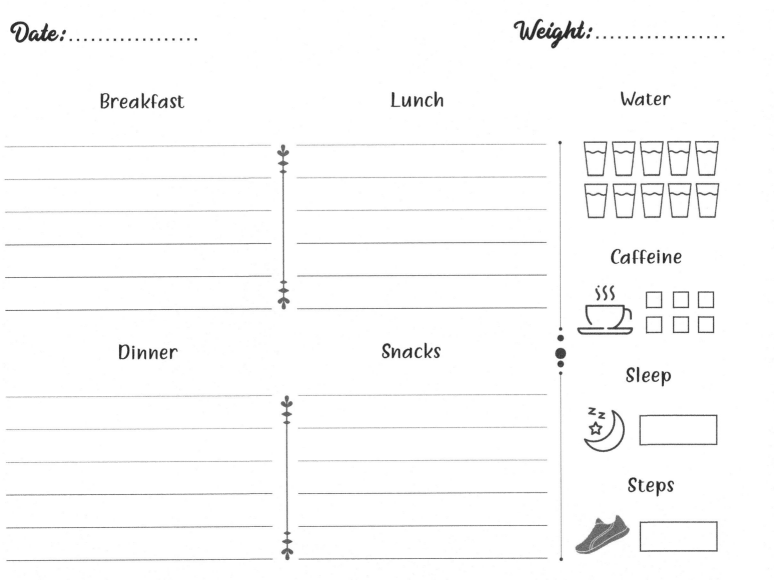

Breakfast

Lunch

Water

Caffeine

Dinner

Snacks

Sleep

Steps

ACTIVITY/EXERCISE	AMOUNT	NOTES

My Mood is

How to make tomorrow better

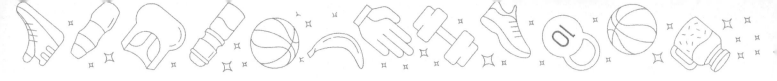

Weekly Check-in

Weekly Goals

☐ _____
_____

☐ _____
_____

☐ _____
_____

Measurements

CHEST	
WAIST	
HIPS	
THIGH	
CALF	
WEIGHT	

Good Habits to Build

_____

_____

_____

_____

_____

Bad Habits to Cut

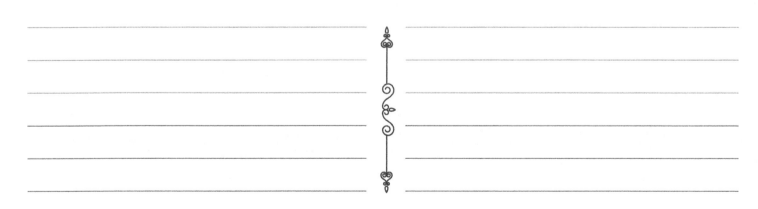

_____

_____

_____

_____

_____

How I'm Feeling

_____

_____

_____

_____

Reasons to keep Going

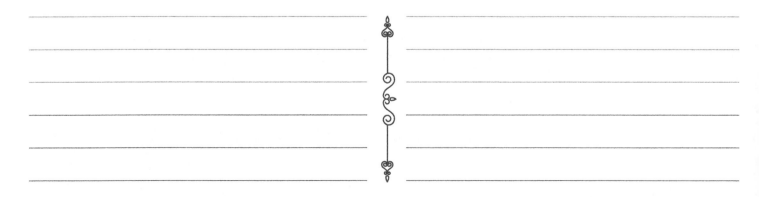

_____

_____

_____

_____

Date: .... Weight: ....

Breakfast

_____
_____
_____
_____
_____

Lunch

_____
_____
_____
_____
_____

Water

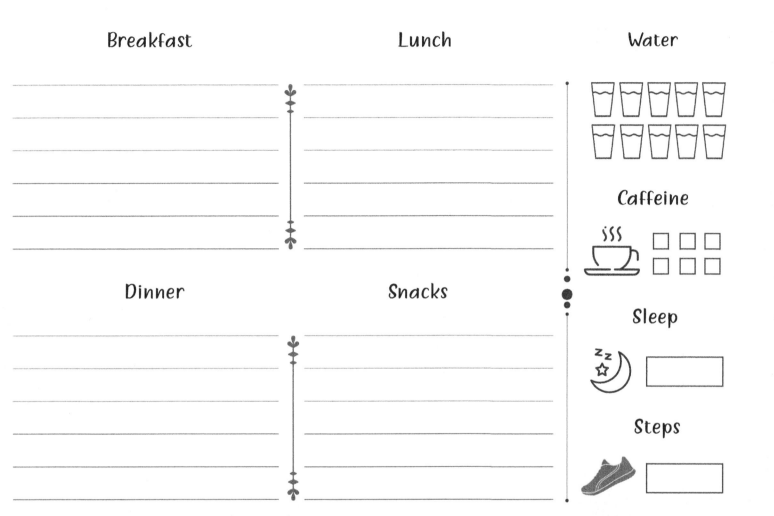

Caffeine

Dinner

_____
_____
_____
_____

Snacks

_____
_____
_____
_____

Sleep

Steps

ACTIVITY/EXERCISE	AMOUNT	NOTES

My Mood is

_____
_____

How to make tomorrow better

_____
_____

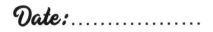

Date:.................

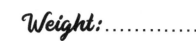

Weight:.................

Breakfast	Lunch	Water

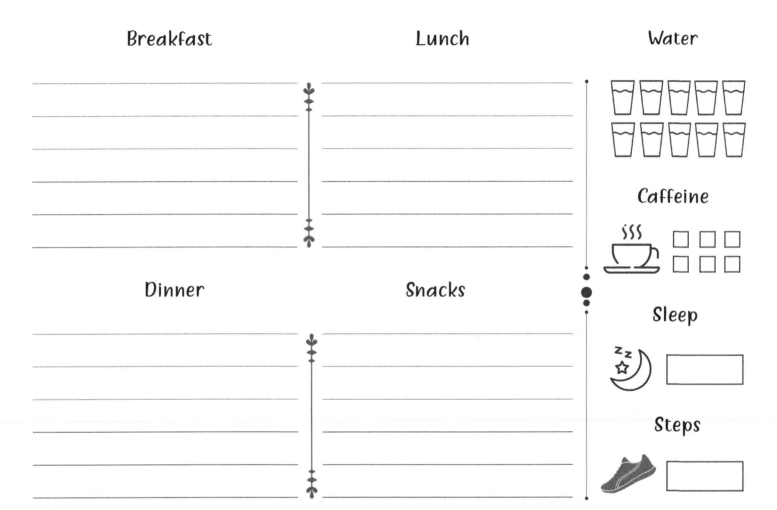

Breakfast
_____
_____
_____
_____
_____

Lunch
_____
_____
_____
_____
_____

Water

Caffeine

Dinner
_____
_____
_____
_____

Snacks
_____
_____
_____
_____

Sleep

Steps

ACTIVITY/EXERCISE	AMOUNT	NOTES

My Mood is
_____
_____
_____

How to make tomorrow better
_____
_____
_____

Date: ....   Weight: ....

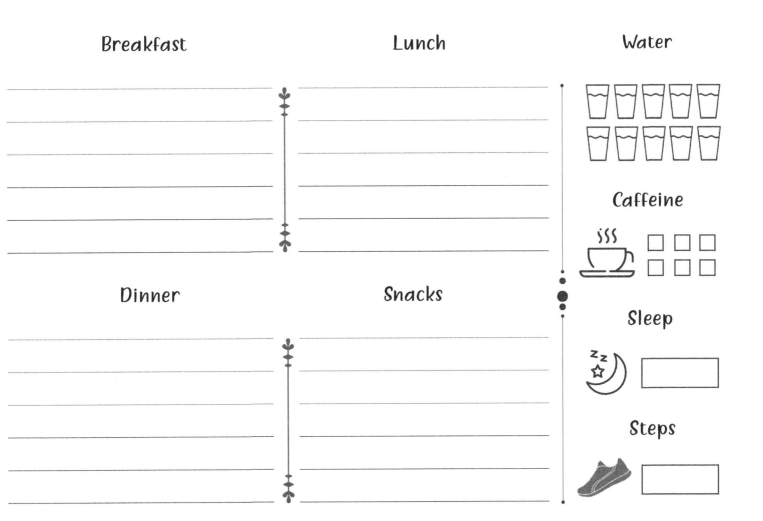

Breakfast

Lunch

Water

Dinner

Snacks

Caffeine

Sleep

Steps

ACTIVITY/EXERCISE	AMOUNT	NOTES

My Mood is

How to make tomorrow better

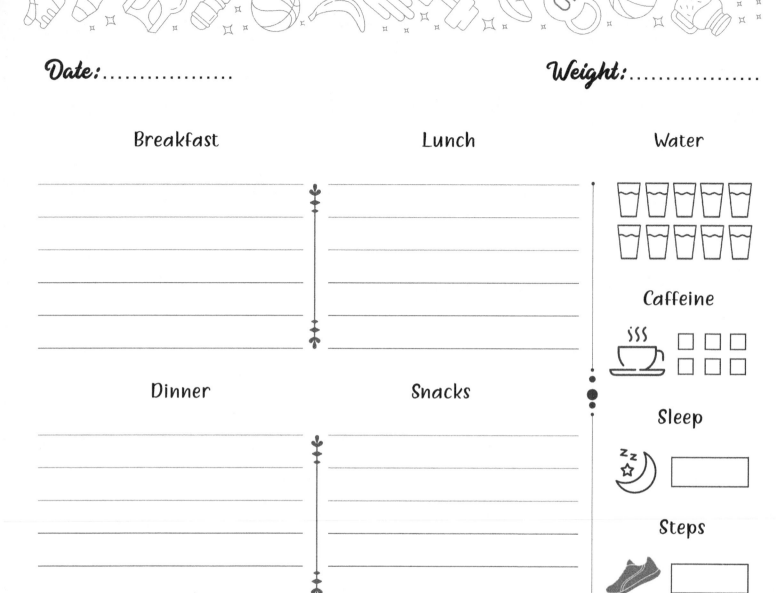

Date:................

Weight:................

Breakfast

_____
_____
_____
_____
_____

Lunch

_____
_____
_____
_____
_____

Water

Caffeine

Dinner

_____
_____
_____
_____
_____

Snacks

_____
_____
_____
_____
_____

Sleep

Steps

ACTIVITY/EXERCISE	AMOUNT	NOTES	

My Mood is

_____
_____

How to make tomorrow better

_____
_____
_____

Date: ....   Weight: ....

Breakfast	Lunch	Water

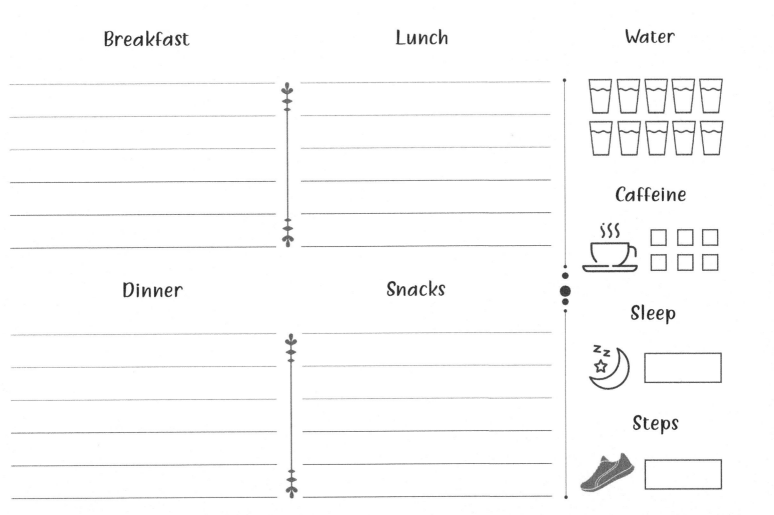

Caffeine

Dinner   Snacks

Sleep

Steps

ACTIVITY/EXERCISE	AMOUNT	NOTES

My Mood is   How to make tomorrow better

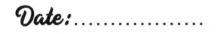

Date: ....   **Weight:** ....

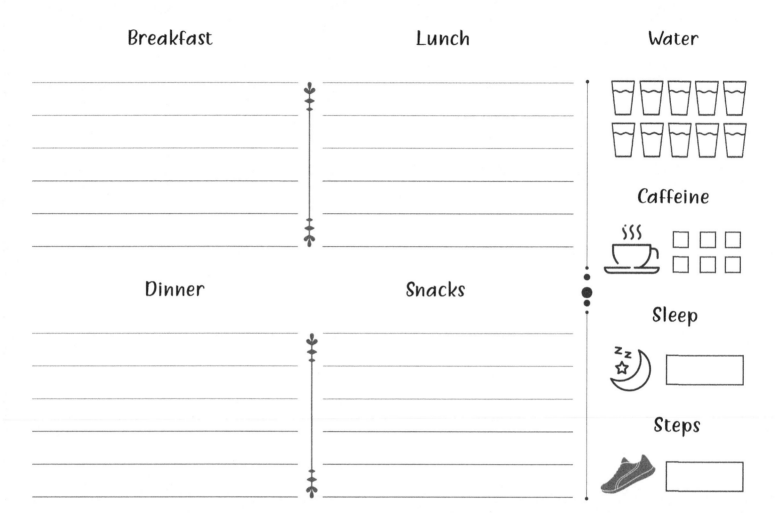

Breakfast	Lunch	Water

Dinner   Snacks   Caffeine

Sleep

Steps

ACTIVITY/EXERCISE	AMOUNT	NOTES

My Mood is	How to make tomorrow better

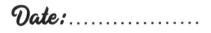

Date: . . . .   **Weight:** . . . .

Breakfast

_____
_____
_____
_____
_____

Lunch

_____
_____
_____
_____
_____

Water

Caffeine

Dinner

_____
_____
_____
_____
_____

Snacks

_____
_____
_____
_____
_____

Sleep

Steps

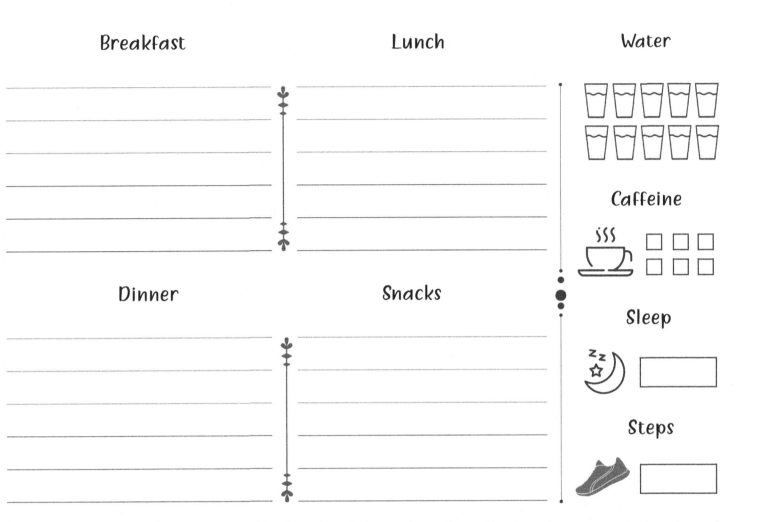

ACTIVITY/EXERCISE	AMOUNT	NOTES

My Mood is

_____
_____

How to make tomorrow better

_____
_____

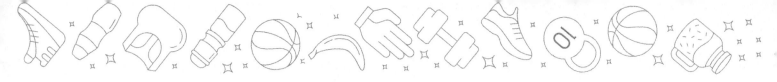

Weekly Check-in

Weekly Goals

- [ ] _____
- [ ] _____
- [ ] _____

Measurements

CHEST	
WAIST	
HIPS	
THIGH	
CALF	
WEIGHT	

Good Habits to Build

_____

_____

_____

_____

Bad Habits to Cut

_____

_____

_____

_____

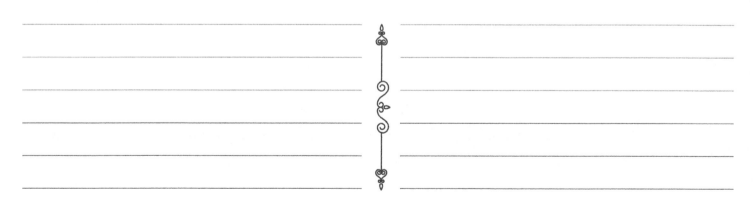

How I'm Feeling

_____

_____

_____

_____

Reasons to keep Going

_____

_____

_____

_____

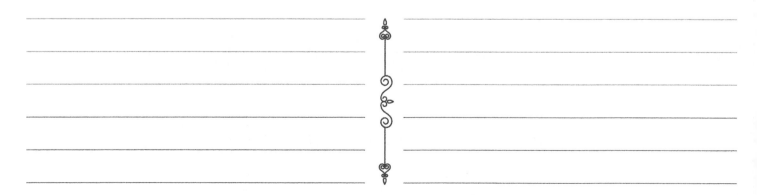

Date: ....

Weight: ....

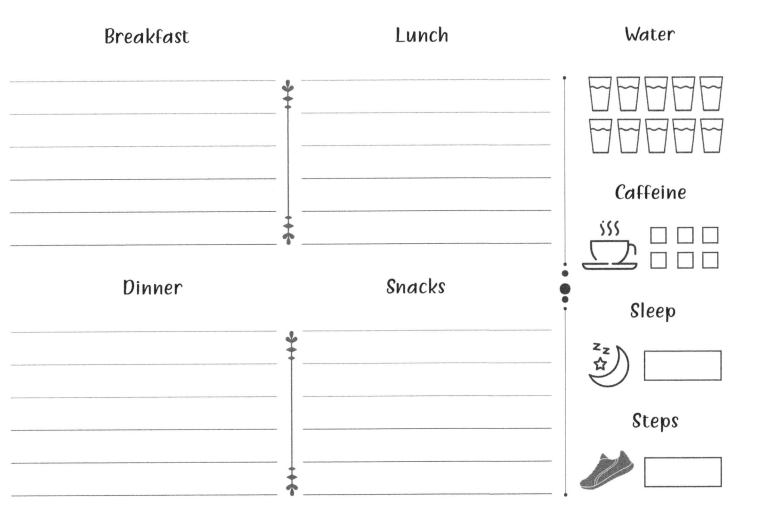

Breakfast

Lunch

Water

Dinner

Snacks

Caffeine

Sleep

Steps

ACTIVITY/EXERCISE	AMOUNT	NOTES

My Mood is

How to make tomorrow better

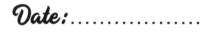

Date: ....   Weight: ....

Breakfast

_____
_____
_____
_____
_____

Lunch

_____
_____
_____
_____
_____

Water

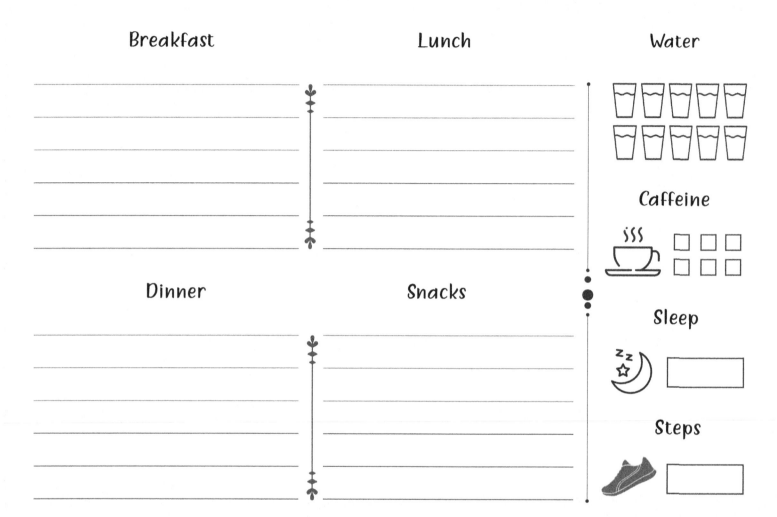

Caffeine

Dinner

_____
_____
_____
_____
_____

Snacks

_____
_____
_____
_____
_____

Sleep

Steps

ACTIVITY/EXERCISE	AMOUNT	NOTES	

My Mood is

_____
_____
_____

How to make tomorrow better

_____
_____
_____

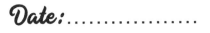

Date: .... **Weight:** ....

Breakfast

Lunch

Water

Dinner

Snacks

Caffeine

Sleep

Steps

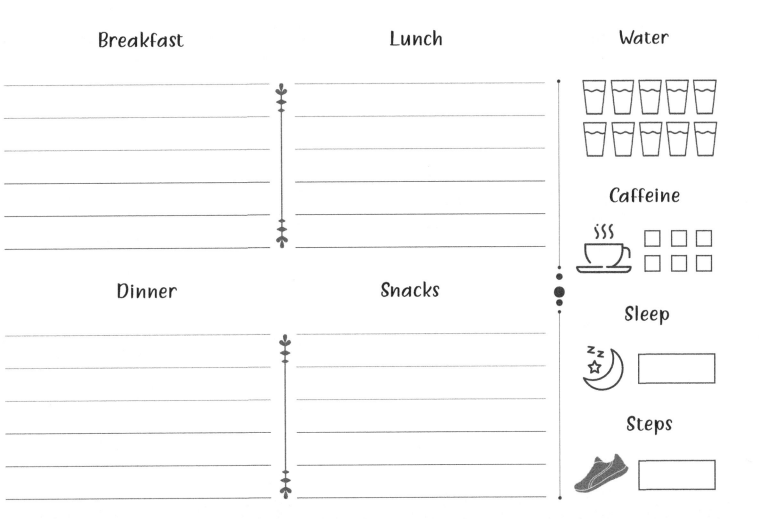

ACTIVITY/EXERCISE	AMOUNT	NOTES

My Mood is

How to make tomorrow better

Date: .... **Weight:** ....

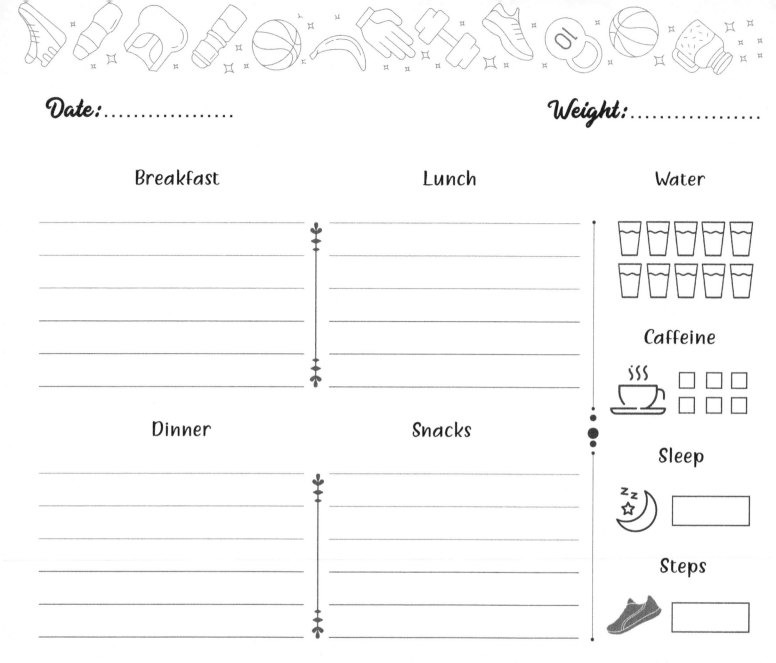

Breakfast

_____
_____
_____
_____
_____

Lunch

_____
_____
_____
_____
_____

Water

Caffeine

Dinner

_____
_____
_____
_____
_____

Snacks

_____
_____
_____
_____
_____

Sleep

Steps

ACTIVITY/EXERCISE	AMOUNT	NOTES

My Mood is

_____
_____

How to make tomorrow better

_____
_____

Date: ....

Weight: ....

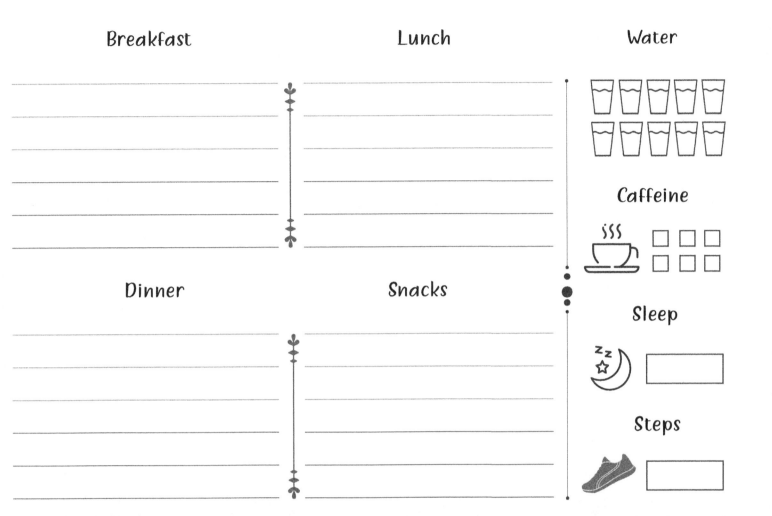

Breakfast

Lunch

Water

Dinner

Snacks

Caffeine

Sleep

Steps

ACTIVITY/EXERCISE	AMOUNT	NOTES

My Mood is

How to make tomorrow better

Date: .... **Weight:** ....

Breakfast
_____
_____
_____
_____
_____

Lunch
_____
_____
_____
_____
_____

Water
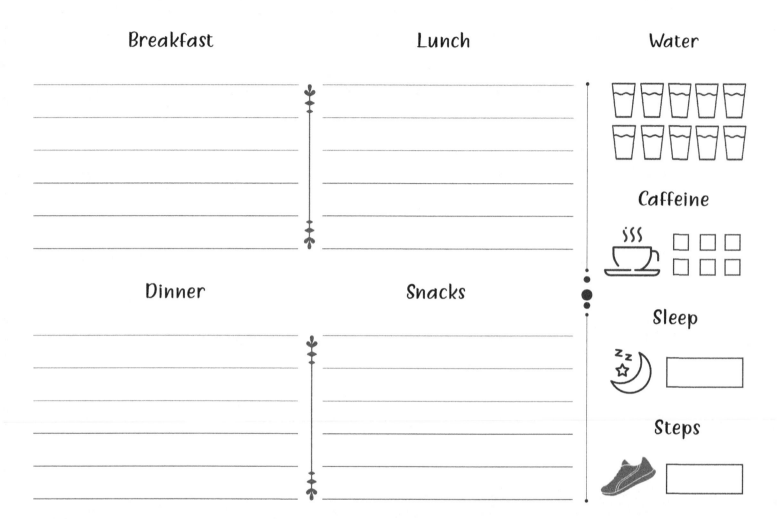

Caffeine

Dinner
_____
_____
_____
_____

Snacks
_____
_____
_____
_____

Sleep

Steps

ACTIVITY/EXERCISE	AMOUNT	NOTES

My Mood is
_____
_____
_____

How to make tomorrow better
_____
_____
_____

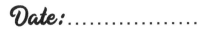

Date: ....   *Weight:* ....

Breakfast

Lunch

Water

Dinner

Snacks

Caffeine

Sleep

Steps

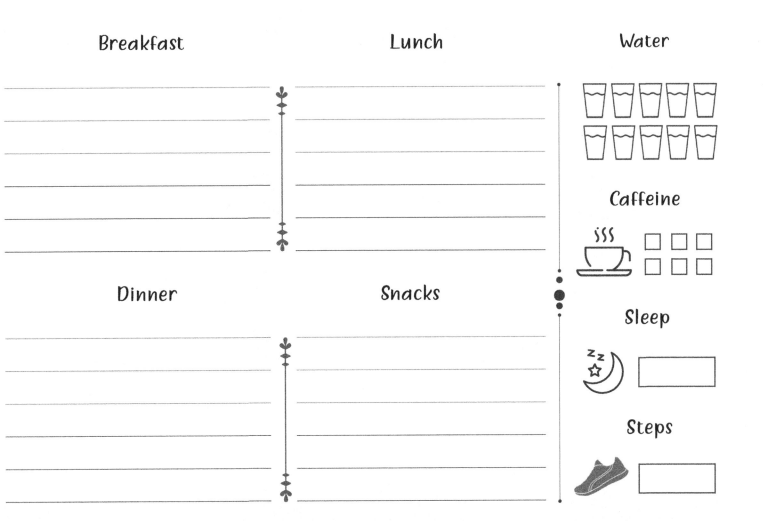

ACTIVITY/EXERCISE	AMOUNT	NOTES

My Mood is

How to make tomorrow better

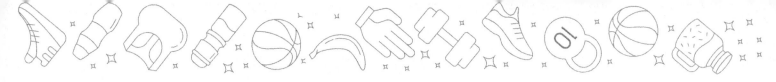

Weekly Check-in

Weekly Goals

☐ _____
_____

☐ _____
_____

☐ _____
_____

Measurements

CHEST	
WAIST	
HIPS	
THIGH	
CALF	
WEIGHT	

Good Habits to Build

_____
_____
_____
_____
_____

Bad Habits to Cut

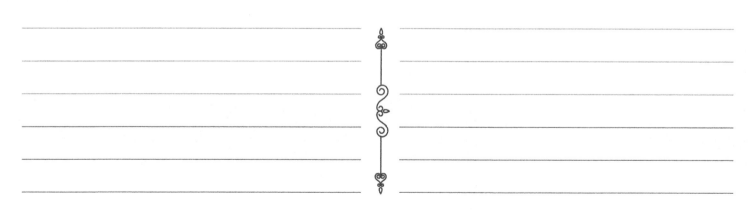

_____
_____
_____
_____
_____

How I'm Feeling

_____
_____
_____
_____

Reasons to keep Going

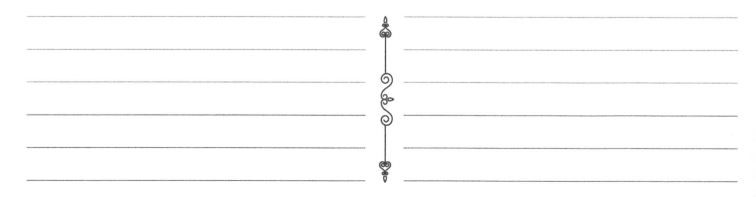

_____
_____
_____
_____

Date:.................   Weight:.................

Breakfast   Lunch   Water

Dinner   Snacks   Caffeine

Sleep

Steps

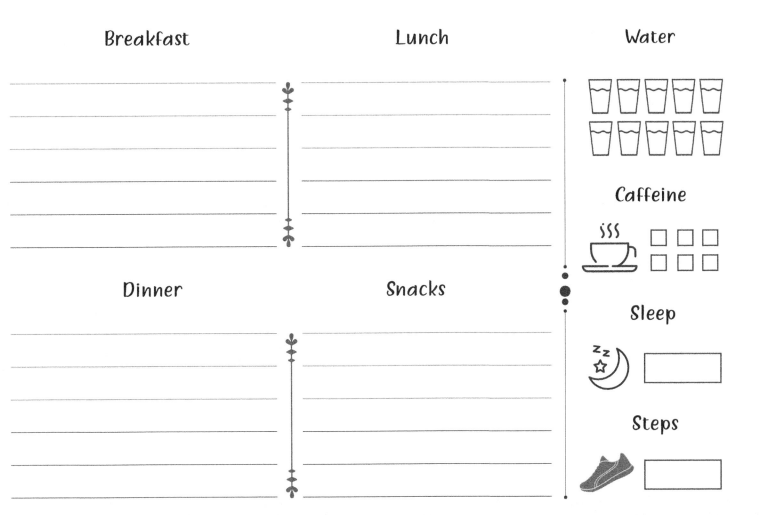

ACTIVITY/EXERCISE	AMOUNT	NOTES

My Mood is   How to make tomorrow better

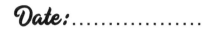

Date: ....   Weight: ....

Breakfast

_____
_____
_____
_____
_____

Lunch

_____
_____
_____
_____
_____

Water

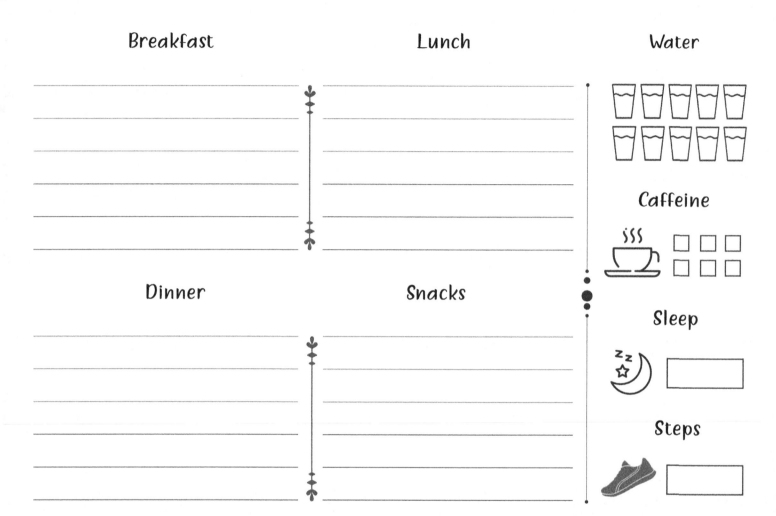

Caffeine

Sleep

Steps

Dinner

_____
_____
_____
_____
_____

Snacks

_____
_____
_____
_____
_____

ACTIVITY/EXERCISE	AMOUNT	NOTES

My Mood is

_____
_____
_____

How to make tomorrow better

_____
_____
_____

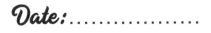

Date:........................ **Weight:**........................

Breakfast

_____
_____
_____
_____
_____
_____

Lunch

_____
_____
_____
_____
_____
_____

Water

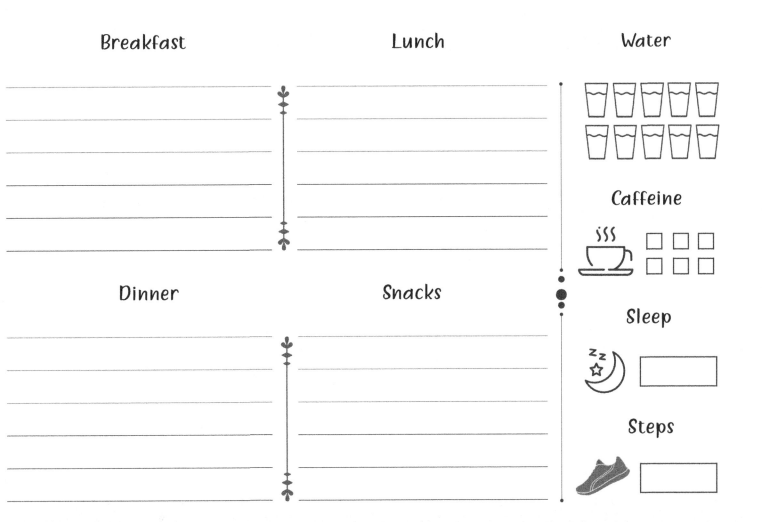

Caffeine

Dinner

_____
_____
_____
_____
_____
_____

Snacks

_____
_____
_____
_____
_____
_____

Sleep

Steps

ACTIVITY/EXERCISE	AMOUNT	NOTES

My Mood is

_____
_____
_____

How to make tomorrow better

_____
_____
_____

Date: .... Weight: ....

Breakfast	Lunch	Water

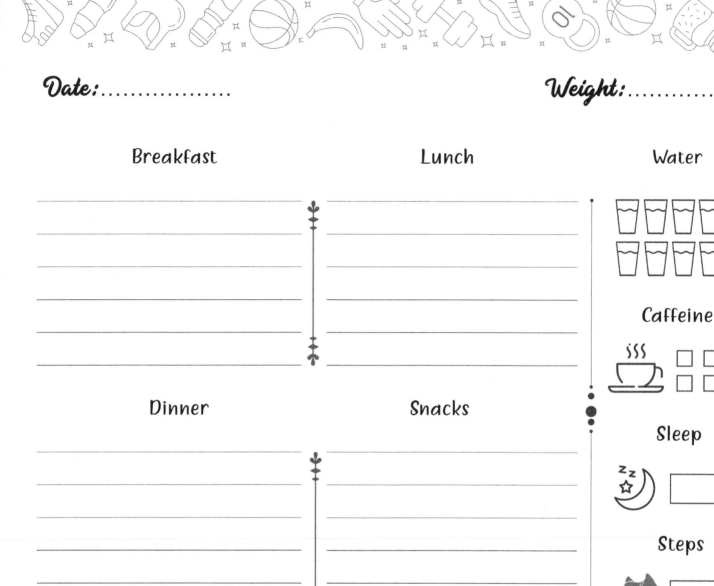

Caffeine

Dinner   Snacks

Sleep

Steps

ACTIVITY/EXERCISE	AMOUNT	NOTES	

My Mood is   How to make tomorrow better

Date: .... **Weight:** ....

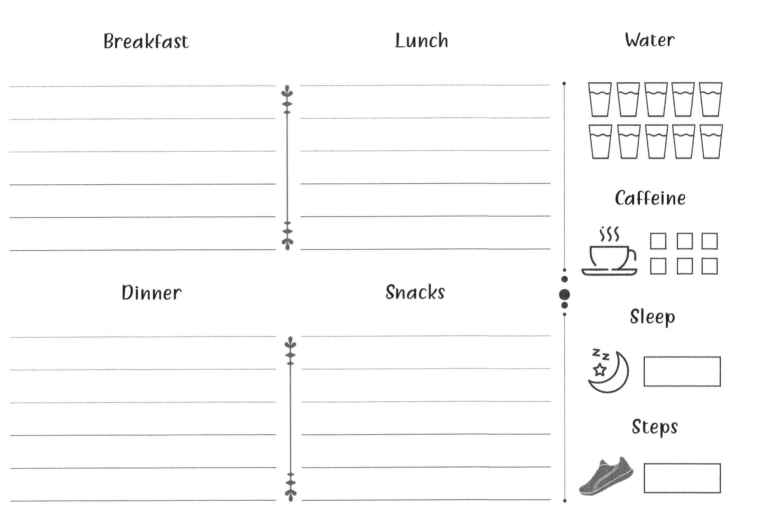

Breakfast

Lunch

Water

Dinner

Snacks

Caffeine

Sleep

Steps

ACTIVITY/EXERCISE	AMOUNT	NOTES

My Mood is

How to make tomorrow better

Date: .... Weight: ....

Breakfast

_____
_____
_____
_____
_____

Lunch

_____
_____
_____
_____
_____

Water

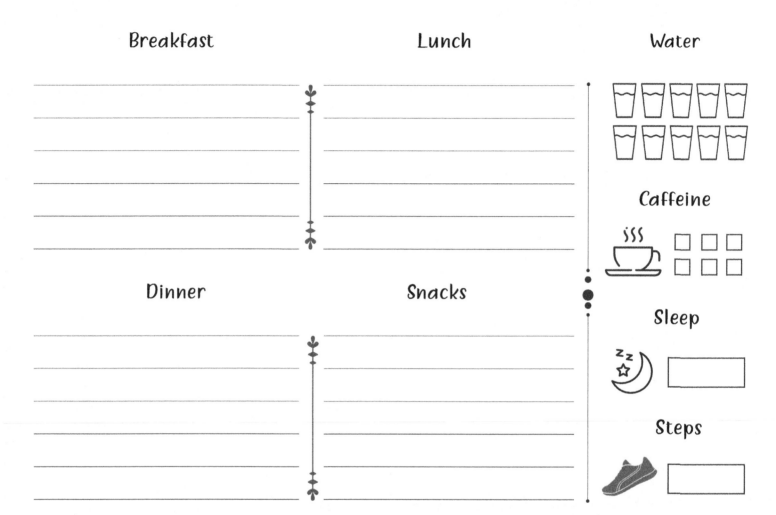

Caffeine

Sleep

Steps

Dinner

_____
_____
_____
_____
_____

Snacks

_____
_____
_____
_____
_____

ACTIVITY/EXERCISE	AMOUNT	NOTES

My Mood is

_____
_____
_____

How to make tomorrow better

_____
_____
_____

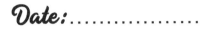

Date: ....   **Weight:** ....

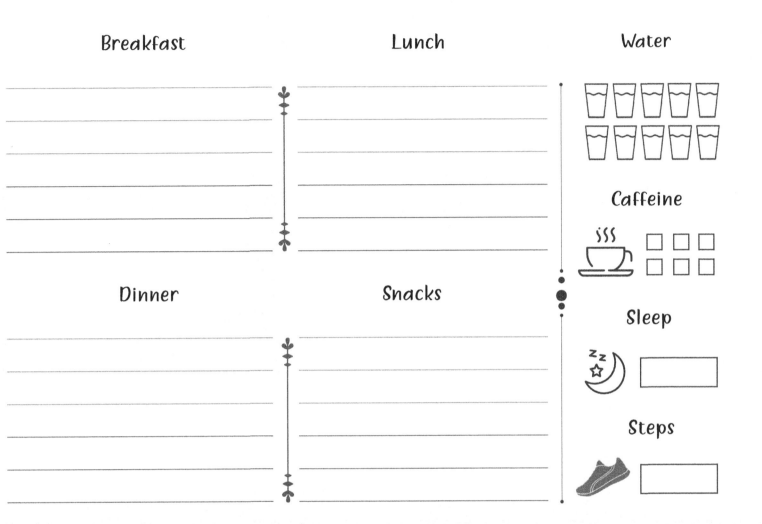

Breakfast

Lunch

Water

Dinner

Snacks

Caffeine

Sleep

Steps

ACTIVITY/EXERCISE	AMOUNT	NOTES

My Mood is

How to make tomorrow better

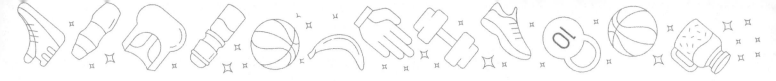

Weekly Check-in

Weekly Goals

- [ ]
_____

- [ ]
_____

- [ ]
_____

Measurements

CHEST	
WAIST	
HIPS	
THIGH	
CALF	
WEIGHT	

Good Habits to Build

_____

_____

_____

_____

_____

Bad Habits to Cut

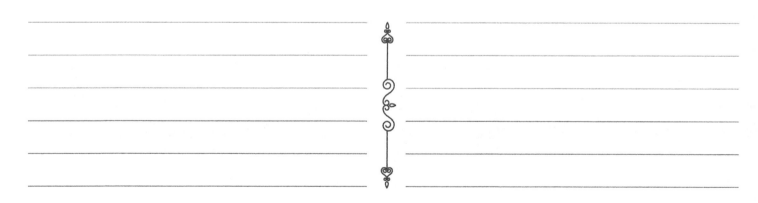

_____

_____

_____

_____

_____

How I'm Feeling

_____

_____

_____

_____

Reasons to keep Going

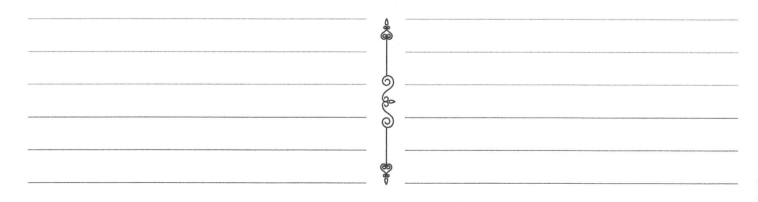

_____

_____

_____

_____

Date:...................   Weight:..................

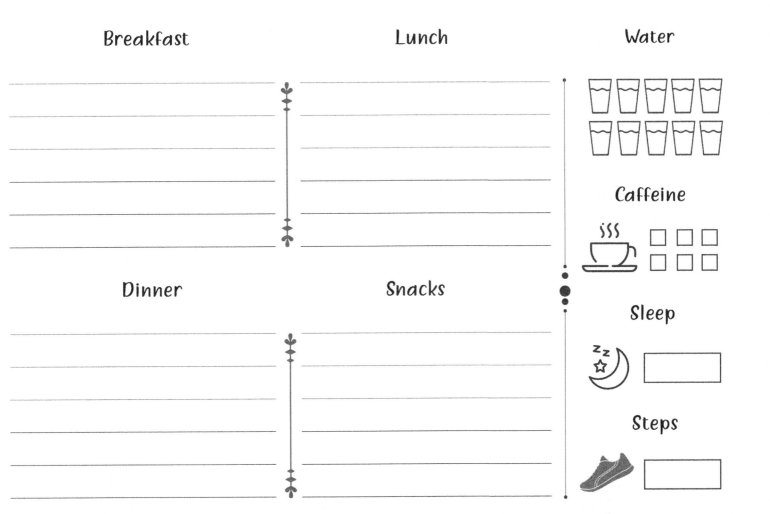

Breakfast

Lunch

Water

Dinner

Snacks

Caffeine

Sleep

Steps

ACTIVITY/EXERCISE	AMOUNT	NOTES

My Mood is

How to make tomorrow better

Date: ....

Weight: ....

Breakfast

Lunch

Water

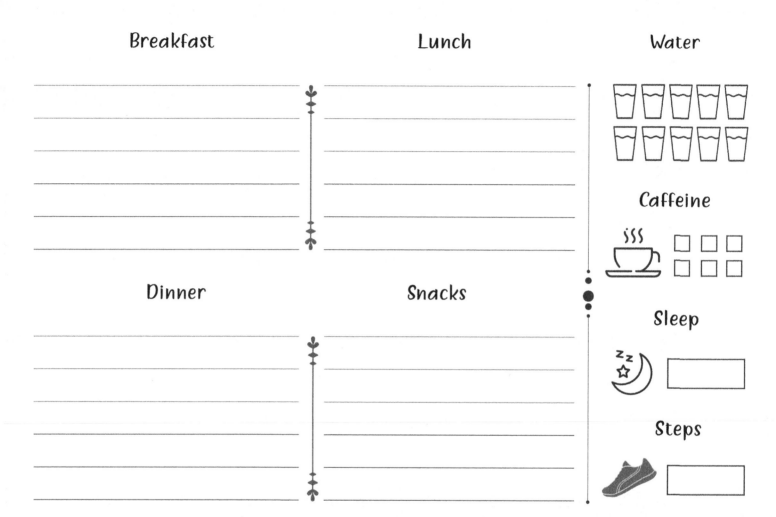

Caffeine

Dinner

Snacks

Sleep

Steps

ACTIVITY/EXERCISE	AMOUNT	NOTES	

My Mood is

How to make tomorrow better

Date: ....

Weight: ....

Breakfast

Lunch

Water

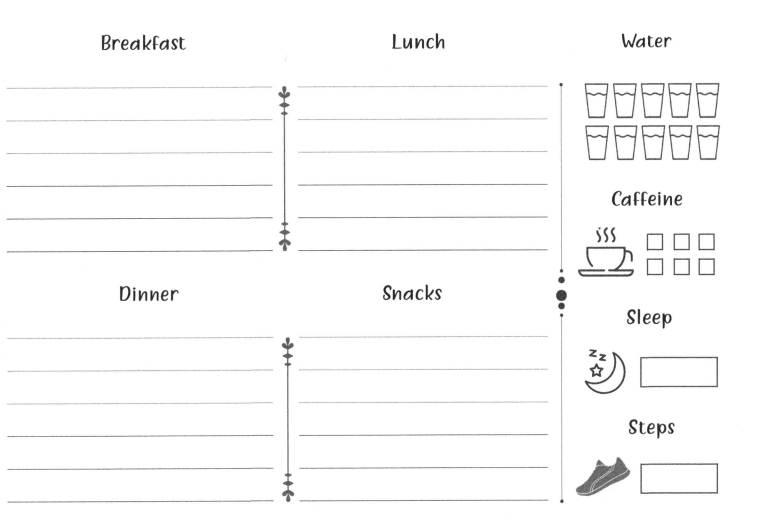

Dinner

Snacks

Caffeine

Sleep

Steps

ACTIVITY/EXERCISE	AMOUNT	NOTES

My Mood is

How to make tomorrow better

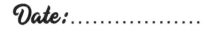

Date: ....

Weight: ....

Breakfast

_____
_____
_____
_____
_____
_____

Lunch

_____
_____
_____
_____
_____
_____

Water

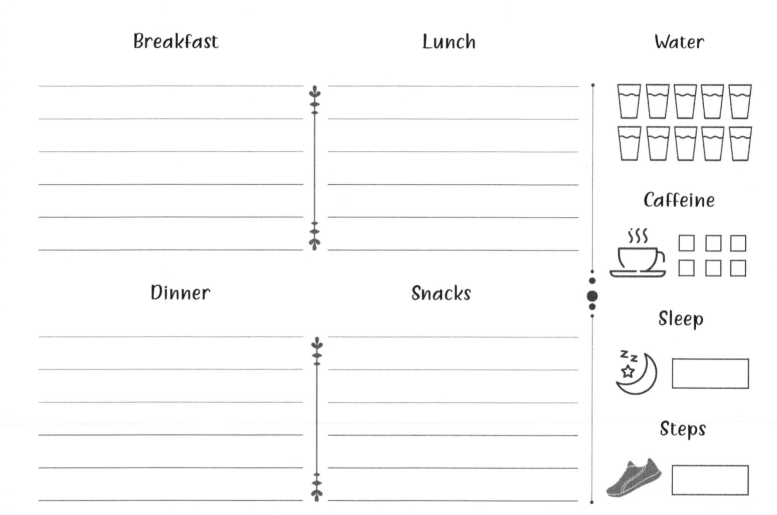

Caffeine

Dinner

_____
_____
_____
_____
_____
_____

Snacks

_____
_____
_____
_____
_____
_____

Sleep

Steps

ACTIVITY/EXERCISE	AMOUNT	NOTES

My Mood is

_____
_____
_____

How to make tomorrow better

_____
_____
_____

Date: .... **Weight:** ....

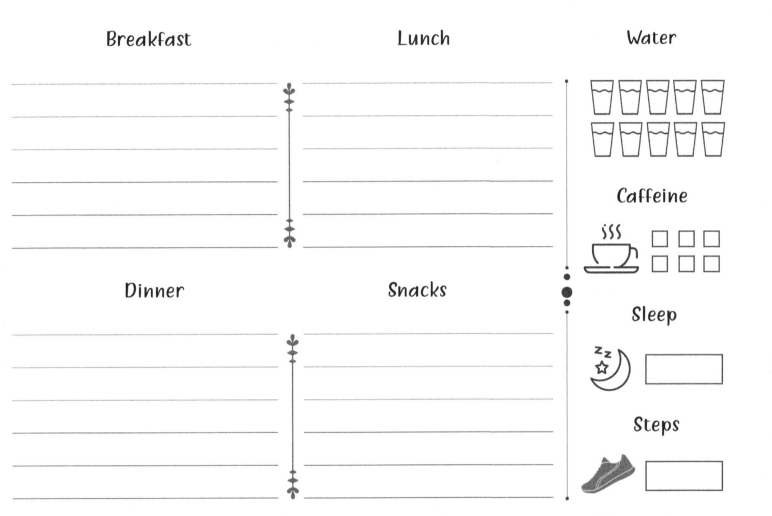

Breakfast

Lunch

Water

Dinner

Snacks

Caffeine

Sleep

Steps

ACTIVITY/EXERCISE	AMOUNT	NOTES

My Mood is

How to make tomorrow better

Date: ....   **Weight:** ....

Breakfast	Lunch	Water

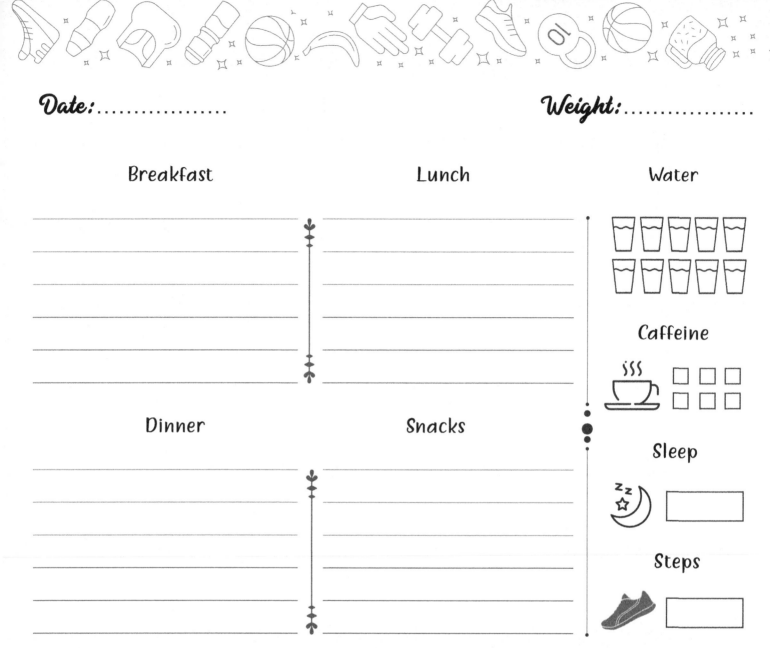

Caffeine

Sleep

Steps

ACTIVITY/EXERCISE	AMOUNT	NOTES

My Mood is	How to make tomorrow better

Date: .... Weight: ....

Breakfast

Lunch

Water

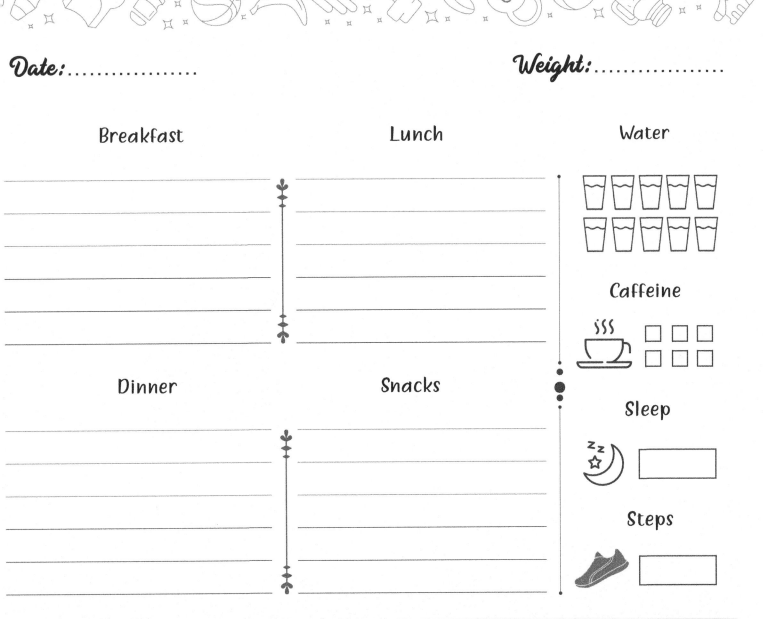

Caffeine

Dinner

Snacks

Sleep

Steps

ACTIVITY/EXERCISE	AMOUNT	NOTES

My Mood is

How to make tomorrow better

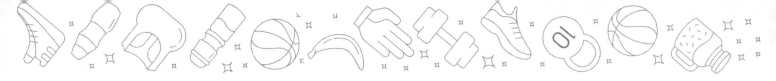

Weekly Check-in

Weekly Goals

- [ ] _____
- [ ] _____
- [ ] _____

Measurements

CHEST	
WAIST	
HIPS	
THIGH	
CALF	
WEIGHT	

Good Habits to Build

Bad Habits to Cut

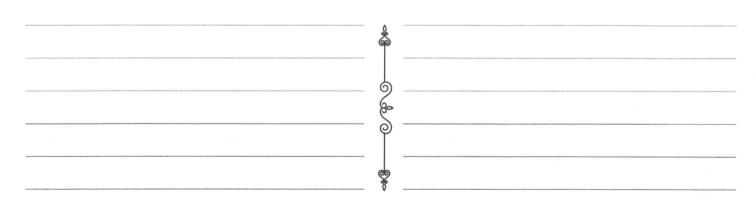

How I'm Feeling

Reasons to keep Going

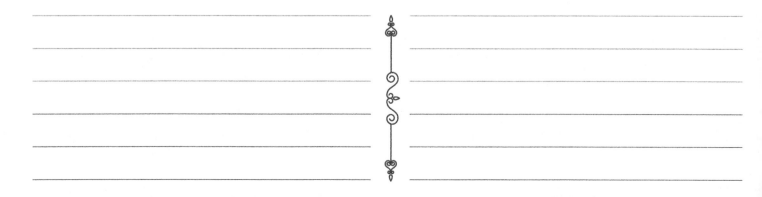

Notes

Notes